CONTRACEPTION
MADE EASY
REVISED EDITION

LAURA PERCY

Specialist Registrar in Community Sexual and Reproductive Health
New Croft Centre, Newcastle upon Tyne, UK

and

DIANA MANSOUR

Consultant in Community Gynaecology and Reproductive Healthcare
New Croft Centre, Newcastle upon Tyne, UK

Scion

© **Scion Publishing Ltd, 2016**

Revised edition published 2016

First edition (ISBN 978 1 907904 30 1) published in 2015

A CIP catalogue record for this book is available from the British Library.

ISBN 978 1 907904 92 9

Scion Publishing Limited

The Old Hayloft, Vantage Business Park, Bloxham Road, Banbury OX16 9UX, UK

www.scionpublishing.com

Important Note from the Publisher

The information contained within this book was obtained by Scion Publishing Ltd from sources believed by us to be reliable. However, while every effort has been made to ensure its accuracy, no responsibility for loss or injury whatsoever occasioned to any person acting or refraining from action as a result of information contained herein can be accepted by the authors or publishers.

Readers are reminded that medicine is a constantly evolving science and while the authors and publishers have ensured that all dosages, applications and practices are based on current indications, there may be specific practices which differ between communities. You should always follow the guidelines laid down by the manufacturers of specific products and the relevant authorities in the country in which you are practising.

Although every effort has been made to ensure that all owners of copyright material have been acknowledged in this publication, we would be pleased to acknowledge in subsequent reprints or editions any omissions brought to our attention.

Registered names, trademarks, etc. used in this book, even when not marked as such, are not to be considered unprotected by law.

Illustrations by Hilary Strickland

Typeset by Phoenix Photosetting, Chatham, Kent, UK

Printed in the UK

Contents

Foreword

As the President of the Faculty of Sexual and Reproductive Healthcare (FSRH) I am often asked about the best 'contraceptive' book to buy. Many want a concise yet complete text that is up to date and covers all the salient areas. I was beginning to think that textbooks were a thing of the past and then *Contraception Made Easy* pops up.

The authors are well known to many. Both have published widely. Dr Laura Percy, a senior community sexual and reproductive health trainee, was the first winner of the Anne Szarewski Memorial prize for clinical practice innovation. Dr Diana Mansour is a Consultant in Community Gynaecology and Reproductive Healthcare and leads the integrated sexual health service in Newcastle upon Tyne. She has been an Honorary Lecturer at the University of Newcastle since 1997 and is the Honorary Treasurer and an Officer for the FSRH.

The authors have brought together current FSRH national guidance and best practice into a neat, clear and succinct handbook and they are to be congratulated for doing this. The introduction states that "this short book provides up-to-date information, often in note form, about the commonly used contraceptive methods available in high resource countries and is aimed at healthcare professionals working in primary, community and secondary services". It does exactly that. I cannot imagine anyone providing women's healthcare not benefiting from having a copy.

Dr Chris Wilkinson, President FSRH
August 2015

About the authors

Dr Laura Percy is a ST6 specialist registrar in Community Sexual and Reproductive Health at the New Croft Clinic in Newcastle upon Tyne. She is the winner of the inaugural Anne Szarewski Journal Memorial Award, and has published several articles on Contraception and Women's Health. She completed her MBBS from the University of Newcastle upon Tyne in 2006, began working in contraception in 2008 and joined the Faculty of Sexual and Reproductive Health's Speciality Training programme in 2012. She has an MSc in Health Education and Health Promotion, and a BSc in Human Biology from King's College, London.

Dr Diana Mansour is a Consultant in Community Gynaecology and Reproductive Healthcare and Head of Sexual Health Services in Newcastle. She has been an Associate Clinical Lecturer at the University of Newcastle since 1997. In addition Dr Mansour is the Honorary Treasurer and an Officer for the Faculty of Sexual and Reproductive Healthcare. Her areas of expertise include acceptability of contraceptive methods, non-contraceptive benefits of contraception, development of long-term methods of contraception, changes in health service provision, medical management of heavy menstrual bleeding, menopause and hormone replacement therapy.

Dr Mansour was the first accredited subspecialty trainee in Community Gynaecology and Reproductive Healthcare of the Royal College of Obstetricians and Gynaecologists. She is first author to over 80 peer-reviewed publications.

Abbreviations

ART	antiretroviral therapy
BMD	bone mineral density
BMI	body mass index
CHC	combined hormonal contraception
CIN	cervical intraepithelial neoplasia
COC	combined oral contraceptive
CTP	combined transdermal patch
CVE	cardiovascular event
CVR	combined vaginal ring
DMPA	depot medroxyprogesterone acetate
DVT	deep vein thrombosis
EC	emergency contraception
EVA	electronic vacuum aspiration
FPA	Family Planning Association
FSH	follicle-stimulating hormone
hCG	human chorionic gonadotrophin
HMB	heavy menstrual bleeding
IBD	inflammatory bowel disease

IMB	intermenstrual bleeding
IUC	intrauterine contraceptive
IUD	intrauterine device
IUS	intrauterine system
IVF	*in vitro* fertilization
LARC	long-acting reversible contraception
LH	luteinizing hormone
LNG	levonorgestrel
MI	myocardial infarction
MIV	minimally invasive vasectomy
MVA	manual vacuum aspiration
NET-EN	norethisterone enanthate
NICE	National Institute for Health and Care Excellence
NSAID	non-steroidal anti-inflammatory drug
NSV	no-scalpel vasectomy
PCB	post-coital bleeding
PE	pulmonary embolism
PEPSE	post-exposure prophylaxis following sexual exposure
PID	pelvic inflammatory disease
POP	progestogen-only pill
RCOG	Royal College of Obstetricians and Gynaecologists
STI	sexually transmitted infection
UKMEC	UK Medical Eligibility Criteria
UPA	ulipristal acetate
UPSI	unprotected sexual intercourse
VTE	venous thromboembolism

Chapter 1
Introduction

1.1 Introduction

This short book provides up-to-date information, often in note form, about the commonly used contraceptive methods available in high resource countries and is aimed at healthcare professionals working in primary, community and secondary services. The book's content is based on guidance from the Faculty of Sexual and Reproductive Healthcare's Clinical Effectiveness Unit and the National Institute for Health and Care Excellence. References will appear at the end of each chapter when specific studies or reviews are mentioned.

Chapter 2, covering the consultation, explores the necessary points to discuss when seeing couples about contraception, including their ideas, concerns and expectations. *Chapter 3* looks in more detail at the provision of contraception to special groups such as young people and those with learning difficulties. Each method will then be examined in turn, with information identifying potential users of the method, how it works, its efficacy, the advantages and disadvantages, how to start and stop the methods (where appropriate) plus the management of troublesome side-effects. The book concludes with two chapters on screening women for asymptomatic sexually transmitted infections (STI) and managing unplanned pregnancies.

1.2 Unplanned pregnancy

Keeping up to date in this field is difficult, especially when contraception is not a special interest of the nurse or doctor. Yet men and women will seek advice from approachable healthcare staff who are non-judgemental and can give non-directional support. Hopefully being better prepared will help couples plan their pregnancies. However, at the current time it is estimated that almost 50% of pregnancies worldwide are unplanned. One in three women from high resource countries experiences an abortion during their lifetime, with a third requiring a repeat procedure (see *Figure 1.1*).

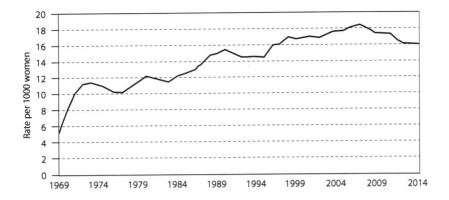

Figure 1.1. Age-standardized abortion rate in women aged 15–44 in England and Wales.

Over 80% of abortions take place in women aged 20 or over, not the teenagers that are so often vilified. At the time of the abortion, at least 60% of women report using a contraceptive method. However, the mostly commonly cited methods are oral contraceptives or condoms, which require correct and consistent use. This high number of unplanned pregnancies may reflect poor contraceptive knowledge in the population. There may be issues related to funding of contraceptive services in primary and community care which limit access to and availability of contraceptive choice. Time pressures during consultations reduce the ability to explore fears and concerns surrounding some methods. This can result in couples choosing a contraceptive that fails to fit their lifestyle, for example an inability to adhere to daily regimens, leading to high typical failure rates for pills, condoms and natural methods when compared with perfect use (*Table 1.1*).

1.3 Provision of contraceptive services

For England and Wales recent years have seen a small fall in the age-standardized abortion rate (see *Figure 1.1*). Many other European countries show a similar trend, but this will only be sustained if there is political commitment to invest in contraceptive choice and easily accessible services. Effective provision of, and access to, contraception improves the health of women and children. Investing in this area of healthcare is cost-effective, with every £1 spent in the UK on contraceptive provision resulting in a cost benefit of £11.09. This rises to £13.42 for every £1 invested in long-acting reversible contraceptive methods (LARCs).

1.4 UK Medical Eligibility Criteria for contraception

Sixteen contraceptive methods are available free at the point of access in the UK and these include:
- emergency contraception
- combined oral contraceptives (COCs), patches, and vaginal rings

Table 1.1. Summary table of contraceptive efficacy – percentage of women experiencing an unintended pregnancy during the first year of typical and perfect use of contraception, and the percentage continuing use of that contraceptive at the end of the first year of use

Contraceptive method	Women experiencing an unintended pregnancy within the first year of use (%)		Women continuing use at 1 year (%)
	Typical use	Perfect use	
No method	85	85	
Spermicides	28	18	42
Fertility awareness-based methods	24		47
Simplified calendar method		5	
Two day method		4	
Ovulation method		3	
Symptothermal method		0.4	
Withdrawal	22	4	46
Sponge			36
Parous women	24	20	
Nulliparous women	12	9	
Condom			
Female	21	5	41
Male	18	2	43
Diaphragm	12	6	57
Combined pill and progestogen-only pill	9	0.3	67
Evra patch	9	0.3	67
NuvaRing	9	0.3	67
Depo-Provera	6	0.2	56
IUDs			
ParaGard (copper T)	0.8	0.6	78
Mirena (LNG)	0.2	0.2	80
Implanon	0.05	0.05	84
Female sterilization	0.5	0.5	100
Male sterilization	0.15	0.10	100

Adapted from Trussell (2012) Contraceptive failure in the United States. *Contraception,* **83**: 397.

- progestogen-only pills (POPs)
- progestogen-only injectables and implants
- copper intrauterine contraceptives (IUDs)
- levonorgestrel intrauterine system (IUS)

- diaphragms, cervical caps
- male and female condoms
- natural fertility awareness advice/kits
- male and female sterilization.

Healthcare professionals may be fully aware of the contraceptive options available to couples but have concerns if certain medical conditions are present. This could deny women at greatest risk of maternal morbidity and mortality highly effective birth control methods. The UK Medical Eligibility Criteria (UKMEC) for contraceptive use is based on guidance from the World Health Organization and has been modified for use in the UK, guiding health professionals towards safer prescribing. The role of the UKMEC is to consider the safety of a method of contraception but not its efficacy with regard to medical conditions and patient characteristics. (See *Appendix* for full details of the UKMEC).

The UKMEC is a comprehensive reference tool for those prescribing contraception. The recommendations within it are based on current research, evidence and expert opinion. It includes four categories of risk applicable to contraceptive methods and these are shown in *Table 1.2*, but can be simply viewed as follows:

- UK Category 1 – no restriction for use
- UK Category 2 – can generally be used but with careful follow-up
- UK Category 3 – not usually recommended but may be used after expert clinical judgement and/or referral to a contraceptive specialist
- UK Category 4 – use poses an unacceptable health risk.

In certain cases, initiation (I) of a contraceptive method is classified differently from continuation (C) of a method:

- initiation – starting a method of contraception by a woman with a specific medical condition
- continuation – continuing with the method already being used by a woman who develops a new medical condition.

Table 1.2. Four categories of risk applicable to contraceptive methods

UK category	Hormonal contraception, IUDs and barrier methods
1	A condition for which there is no restriction for the use of the contraceptive method.
2	A condition where the advantages of using the method generally outweigh the theoretical or proven risks.
3	A condition where the theoretical or proven risks usually outweigh the advantages of using the method. Provision of this method requires expert clinical judgement and/or referral to a specialist contraceptive provider because use of the method is not usually recommended unless other methods are not available or not acceptable.
4	A condition which represents an unacceptable health risk if the contraceptive method is used.

Adapted from the Faculty of Sexual and Reproductive Healthcare's UKMEC for contraception, with kind permission.

There may be an unacceptable risk for a particular method because a medical condition adversely affects the contraceptive method or vice versa.

The UKMEC have recently been updated (2016) and the order in which the methods are presented in the summary document (see *Appendix*) has changed. Long-acting reversible methods of contraception (LARC) are presented first, followed by medium and then shorter-acting methods. Several new medical conditions have been added, including history of bariatric surgery, organ transplant, cardiomyopathy, arrhythmias (AF and long QT syndrome) and rheumatoid arthritis (these additional conditions are highlighted in the *Appendix*). Furthermore, advice for postpartum CHC use has been expanded, including incorporation of VTE risk. The 2016 UKMEC no longer give advice on drug interactions with contraception and recommend resources such as the FSRH, BNF or using online drug information checkers.

In this table, the numbers always refer to the UK Category of risk and in some instances the risk level is different at initiation (I) and continuation (C). The UKMEC should be used as a guide but should not replace clinical judgement. For a summary of the UKMEC see *Appendix*.

References

Bayer HealthCare (2013) *Contraception Atlas 2013*
[http://theagc.org.uk/wp-content/uploads/2013/08/Contraception-Atlas-2013-FINAL.pdf – accessed April 2016]

Department of Health (2015) *Abortion statistics, England and Wales: 2015*
[www.gov.uk/government/statistics/report-on-abortion-statistics-in-england-and-wales-for-2015 – accessed June 2016]

NICE (2014) Clinical guideline 30: *Long-acting reversible contraception* (update)
[www.nice.org.uk/guidance/cg30 – accessed April 2016]

Trussell J. (2011) *Contraceptive efficacy*. In Hatcher, R.A., *et al.* Contraceptive Technology: Twentieth Revised Edition. New York, NY: Ardent Media.
[www.contraceptivetechnology.org/wp-content/uploads/2013/09/CTFailureTable.pdf – accessed April 2016]

UKMEC (2016) *UK Medical Eligibility Criteria for Contraceptive Use*
[www.fsrh.org/standards-and-guidance/uk-medical-eligibility-criteria-for-contraceptive-use/ – accessed June 2016]

Chapter 2
The contraception consultation

2.1 Introduction

The primary aim of the contraception consultation is to enable women to choose the most suitable and acceptable method of birth control for their lifestyle.

A detailed history will help in determining which of the sixteen available methods can be used safely. Furthermore, taking a careful sexual history provides an opportunity for risk assessment, screening for infection and health promotion.

A variety of consultation models exist. They act as aids to help in the development of consultation skills with the aim of generating a patient-centred discussion. Their emphasis is on shared decision making and active participation by both parties. The contraception consultation could be based around any of these models. We suggest the Calgary–Cambridge approach, illustrated in *Figure 2.1*, which offers a useful framework and will be used throughout this book to provide a basic structure for the consultation.

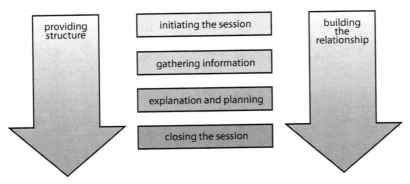

Figure 2.1. Calgary–Cambridge consultation model.

2.2 Initiating the session

This can be divided into two components:
- Establishing initial rapport:
  - greeting the patient
  - introducing yourself.
- Identifying the reason for the consultation:
  - this is ideally undertaken through the use of open questions, for example, *"How can I help you today?"* or *"What would you like to discuss?"*
  - the answers may range from specific requests for a particular method of contraception to the more complex "I need contraception but everything I have tried causes me problems"
  - supporting patients to set the agenda focuses the consultation on the patient's needs and helps to establish rapport.

2.3 Gathering information

- Explore the patient's narrative through a progression from open to closed questions, with active listening.
- An empathetic, non-judgemental approach with appropriate use of summaries or clarifying statements is often beneficial.
- Enable the patient to indicate their ideas, concerns and expectations.
  - **Ideas** – methods of contraception they have considered or previously used; this may include asking about problems encountered with previous methods, why previous contraception was stopped, or what they liked or disliked about previous choices.
  - **Concerns** – for example, worries about side-effects or perceptions about particular methods; this also provides an opportunity to myth bust about contraceptive methods, for example, "pills" cause weight gain and intrauterine devices or systems cannot be used by women who have not had children.
  - **Expectations** – for example, true efficacy, acceptable side-effects.
  - Future plans – would becoming pregnant be a disaster, are there plans to start a family or have another child in the near future?
- By using this approach one can easily determine acceptable methods and those which would be less likely to suit an individual (see *Figure 2.2*).
- Subsequently, a review of a patient's past medical, medication, family and social histories can be used to assess medical suitability for various methods. A detailed summary of the medical history is outlined in *Box 2.1*.
  - This history can be used to determine if there are any contraindications to a particular method of contraception through the application of the UK Medical Eligibility Criteria (UKMEC) – see *Appendix*.
  - A brief review of medical history is often of benefit at each new attendance to ensure circumstances have not changed. If a new medical condition has developed or medication has been initiated or changed, continuation of a patient's chosen method may be inappropriate.

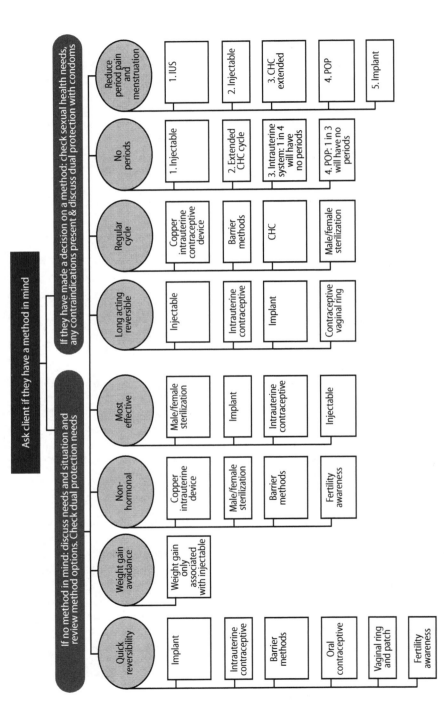

Figure 2.2. Decision tree for contraceptive options.

Box 2.1. Medical history taking in a contraceptive consultation

Age

Gynaecological history

Menstrual cycle details

- Last menstrual period (normal or not)
- Length of cycle (longest and shortest)
- Regularity
- Bleeding irregularities – presence of intermenstrual bleeding (IMB) or post-coital bleeding (PCB), their frequency, duration, and associated symptoms such as pain
- Heavy menstrual bleeding (HMB) or dysmenorrhoea

History of gynaecological conditions

- Ovarian cysts
- Endometriosis
- Pelvic infection

Cervical screening history, if appropriate

Obstetric history

- Previous pregnancies – planned and unplanned
- Number of children, mode of delivery and problems during pregnancy
- Is she breast-feeding?
- Miscarriages
- Ectopic pregnancies
- Abortions

Sexual history

- Any sexual problems?
- Symptoms of sexually transmitted infection (STI) including dysuria, change in vaginal discharge, abdominal pain, skin changes/rash
- Number of sexual partners in last 6 months/recent change in partner
- Condom use

Past medical history

- Epilepsy
- Diabetes
- Hypertension
- Cardiovascular disease
- Venous thromboembolism
- Cerebrovascular disease
- Migraine with or without aura

Medication

- Liver enzyme inducers, e.g. carbamazepine, St. John's wort
- Anti-epileptics
- Herbal remedies/over-the-counter medications

Allergies

Family history – including age at diagnosis and relation to patient

- Myocardial infarction (MI)
- Cardiovascular event (CVE)
- Venous thromboembolism (VTE)
- Breast cancer
- Ovarian cancer

Social history

- Smoking – amount per week
- Alcohol usage – amount per week
- Domestic violence – physical or emotional
- Female genital mutilation

2.4 Explanation and planning

This section of the consultation ideally incorporates the provision of information about available methods including mechanism of action, efficacy, risks, side-effects, and advantages and disadvantages, leading to a shared decision about which method to commence.

- There are a number of possible approaches to take:
  - Each method could be briefly discussed followed by a more detailed discussion of those the patient is most interested in trying; this can be very time-consuming.
  - Alternatively, a good starting point could be to discuss the methods the patient is interested in and then expand on others as needed.
  - Some clinicians start by asking the patient what they know already about individual methods and then build on this foundation. For example, many patients are using online tools such as the 'My contraception tool' found on the websites of the FPA (www.fpa.org.uk/contraception-help/my-contraception-tool) and Brook (www.brook.org.uk/our-services/category/my-contraception-tool).
  - Finally, ask open questions such as *"Apart from preventing a pregnancy, what else would you like your contraceptive method to achieve or help with, such as, to help with period pain or skin problems?"*.
- Ideally information should be provided in small chunks, with regular checks of understanding and at a level appropriate to the individual attending the clinic.
- Practically, the most important aspects to ensure an individual understands about their chosen method are:
  - How to use the method, including missed doses and circumstances when a method will not be effective; for example, vomiting when taking the combined oral contraceptive (COC).
  - How long before it becomes effective.
  - Its benefits, risks and side-effects.
  - Safety-netting to ensure that individuals know when to seek help.
  - Provision of high quality written information, such as FPA leaflets, can be useful both during the consultation and for women to have as a reference at home.
- There are a number of options when starting to use a contraceptive, including:
  - Waiting until the individual's next period before starting contraception.
  - 'Quick starting' – starting contraception at the time a women requests it. This is ideal for the combined hormonal methods, progestogen-only pill (POP) or the implant. *Box 2.2* contains a check list for 'quick starting' contraception if a pregnancy cannot be excluded.
  - Using a bridging contraceptive method until the chosen form of birth control can be commenced, for example, using the POP until pregnancy can be excluded or until an appointment can be arranged to undertake an IUS fitting. This may require explanation of where an individual can obtain their chosen contraceptive if it is not available in your service/practice.
- Discussion regarding risk of STI, advice on safer sexual practices including additional use of condoms, and the offer of STI testing is an important component of a contraception choices consultation.

- o Offer chlamydia and gonorrhoea testing through self-taken vaginal swabs along with blood tests for HIV and syphilis (see *Chapter 14* for more details).
- o Provide information about local condom distribution schemes.
- The contraception consultation provides an opportunity to make enquiry about a history and/or potential risk of female genital mutilation. If the occurrence of FGM or potential risk is identified, national and local pathways should be followed.

Box 2.2. Checklist for 'quick starting' contraception (FSRH, 2010)

If the risk of pregnancy cannot reasonably be excluded, the contraceptive provider should ensure that the woman is:

- likely to continue to be at risk of pregnancy or that she has expressed a preference to begin contraception immediately.
- aware that there is a possibility of pregnancy.
- informed that there is a theoretical risk from fetal exposure to contraceptive hormones but most evidence indicates no harm.
- aware that pregnancy cannot be excluded until she has had a pregnancy test, no sooner than 3 weeks after the last episode of unprotected sexual intercourse.
- provided with a pregnancy testing kit or informed of alternative options for pregnancy testing, including local providers for free testing.
- given advice on additional contraceptive precautions.
- offered a supply of condoms or informed of local providers of condoms.
- advised to return if there are any concerns or problems with her contraception.

2.5 Closing the session

- This provides an opportunity to summarize the session briefly and clarify final choice of method of contraception.
- Follow-up arrangements should be made appropriate to the method selected.
- Safety-nets should be established, with information provided about when to seek help and how to access support if there are any queries or concerns when the clinic or surgery is closed.

2.6 Summary

The contraception consultation is a rewarding and challenging undertaking. It incorporates clinician and patient agendas and, ideally, both are addressed resulting in a satisfactory outcome. The provision of accurate, up-to-date and applicable information empowers women to choose the method they would like. This increases the chance of ongoing and correct use, not to mention patient satisfaction.

EXAMPLE

A 21 year old woman with a history of migraine attends requesting contraception.

Consider what questions you need to ask and which contraceptive options would be appropriate.

1. It is important to determine the nature of the migraine – is it migraine and is there an aura that occurs before the onset of the headache?
2. Take a full gynaecological, obstetric, medical and surgical history along with medication, social and family history.
3. If migraine with aura is identified, combined hormonal contraception (CHC) is contraindicated, but all other methods could be offered. Explain why CHC is contraindicated – associated with an increased risk of stroke in women with migraine with aura.
4. Discuss the most suitable methods (progestogen-only methods, barrier methods and intrauterine devices).
5. Discussion includes mechanism of action, benefits, risks and side-effects, efficacy and time until the method becomes effective.
6. If the selected method is not immediately available, suggest a bridging method and arrange referral/appointment to have the method fitted, as appropriate.

References

FSRH (2010) *Quick Starting Contraception*. Clinical effectiveness unit.
[www.fsrh.org/documents/ceuguidancequickstartingcontraception/ – accessed June 2016]

Home Office (2015) *Mandatory Reporting of Female Genital Mutilation* – procedural information.
[www.gov.uk/government/uploads/system/uploads/attachment_data/file/469448/FGM-Mandatory-Reporting-procedural-info-FINAL.pdf – accessed March 2016]

Kurtz, S.M., Silverman, J.D. and Draper, J. (1998) *Teaching and Learning Communication Skills in Medicine*. Oxford: Radcliffe Medical Press.

UKMEC (2016) *UK Medical Eligibility Criteria for Contraceptive Use*
[www.fsrh.org/standards-and-guidance/uk-medical-eligibility-criteria-for-contraceptive-use/ – accessed June 2016]

Chapter 3
Special groups

There are several groups for whom the provision of contraception can present additional challenges. This chapter considers these challenges in more detail and explores contraceptive provision for young people, those over 40 years, couples with physical disabilities or learning difficulties, HIV-positive women, and women with inflammatory bowel disease (IBD), cardiovascular disease or drug interactions.

3.1 Young people

'Young people' normally refers to those under the age of 18 years. For those over 16 years an ability to consent is assumed unless there are additional factors such as learning disability. For those under 16 years an assessment of competence to consent is undertaken.

3.1.1 Consent

For an individual to be deemed able to consent they would be expected to demonstrate an ability to understand, retain and weigh up the information given to them regarding the intervention and then communicate their decision. Fraser guidelines can provide a useful outline for this process and they are summarized in *Box 3.1*; they are applicable to England, Wales and Northern Ireland. In Scotland the only criterion which needs to be met is that the individual understands the nature of the treatment offered and the consequences of that treatment.

At the beginning of the consultation there should be a discussion regarding the need to breach confidentiality if concerns arise.

3.1.2 Other issues

- For all consultations involving young and/or vulnerable individuals an assessment of potential abuse or exploitation is recommended.

Box 3.1. Fraser guidelines
- The young person understands the professional's advice.
- The young person cannot be persuaded to inform their parents.
- The young person is likely to begin or to continue having sex with or without contraceptive treatment.
- Unless the young person receives contraceptive treatment, their physical and/or mental health is likely to suffer.
- The young person's best interests require them to receive contraceptive advice or treatment with or without parental consent.

- Age is not a limiting factor for contraceptive choice, and a comprehensive history and discussion of available options enables young people to make an informed choice.
- Research suggests that the contraceptive choices made by young people are influenced by multiple factors including efficacy, safety, side-effect profile, invasiveness, ease of use and their knowledge of the method.
- In addition, young people often have particular areas of concern, for example, weight gain or acne, which if elicited and discussed may improve the acceptability of, and compliance with, a chosen method.
- Given the higher incidence of STIs in young people a discussion regarding sexual health, STI prevention and the offer of STI testing, where appropriate, is good practice.

3.2 Women over 40 years of age

- Age alone is not a contraindication to the use of any method of contraception. The final decision is often based on the interplay between medical conditions, menstrual history and the acceptability of a method to a given individual.
- The average age of the menopause is 51–52 years. Women using non-hormonal contraceptives can be advised to stop their contraceptive after 1 year of amenorrhoea if they are over 50 years of age and after 2 years if under 50 years.
- Assessment of follicle-stimulating hormone (FSH) level is generally of limited benefit in peri-menopausal women and should not be relied upon in women under 50 years of age. Levels are affected by CHCs and vary from day to day.
- Checking FSH in CHC users is only of benefit if the CHC is discontinued for a minimum of 6 weeks prior to testing. If FSH levels are then >30 IU/L on two occasions at least 2 weeks apart then it is likely that women over the age of 50 are menopausal and contraception can be stopped after a further 1 year.
- Peri-menopausal women taking CHCs may develop flushes and sweats in the hormone-free interval. Reducing the hormone-free interval to 4 days or using an extended regimen may alleviate these symptoms.
- For women over the age of 40, the lowest possible dose of oestrogen (<30 mcg or an oestradiol-containing CHC) is recommended. Furthermore, at the age of 50 years a CHC is normally changed to a progestogen-only method.
- Women who are amenorrhoeic using progestogen-only methods of contraception can continue until 55 years of age.

- For those women using a progestogen-only injectable, the advice is to change to an alternative method by the age of 50 years. However, if a woman wishes to continue with the progestogen-only injectable and understands the risk and benefits, particularly with regard to their skeletal health, the risk is not unacceptable and use of the progestogen-only injectable contraceptive may continue.
- Any copper intrauterine device inserted after the age of 40 can be used until contraception is no longer required, or 1 year after the menopause in the over 50s.
- A levonorgestrel intrauterine system (containing 52 mg) inserted after the age of 45 is effective for 7 years. After this time if the woman is amenorrhoeic it can continue to be used until she is 55.

3.3 HIV-positive women

- Currently there are no evidence-based guidelines on contraception in HIV-positive women and so pragmatic discussions focusing on practicality and patient choice are advisable.
- Prevention of transmission of HIV and other STIs is routinely discussed with HIV-positive individuals and safe sex promoted.
- Consistent condom use along with an additional contraceptive method (known as dual protection) is recommended for HIV-positive women to prevent pregnancy and reduce horizontal transmission. Consistent use of a condom at each occurrence of sex in serodiscordant couples reduces the risk of HIV transmission by 80%. Condoms lubricated with the spermicide nonoxynol-9 (the only spermicide available in the UK) are not recommended because the spermicide can cause mucosal irritation and has been shown to increase the risk of HIV transmission.
- All methods of contraception are suitable for women who are not on antiretroviral therapy (ART).
- HIV drug interaction websites such as www.hiv-druginteractions.org provide a valuable reference for assessing potential drug interaction prior to commencing contraception.
- Many of the drugs which form part of ART interact with combined oral contraceptives, progestogen-only pills and contraceptive implants.
- The efficacy of the injectable contraceptive, intrauterine systems and intrauterine devices is not affected by ART.
- HIV infection appears to be associated with reduced bone density and individuals with HIV more commonly have osteopenia than the general population. In addition, some ART medications such as tenofovir reduce bone density. Research suggesting a link between bone loss and protease inhibitors is contradictory.
- Progestogen-only injectable contraception may be used in women with HIV including those on ART following discussion of the risks and benefits. In these circumstances a baseline bone density scan may be appropriate prior to starting this method of contraception.
- A recent meta-analysis (Ralph *et al.*, 2015) indicated that women using the progestogen-only injectable contraceptive have a 31–40% increased risk of acquiring HIV compared to users of other methods of contraception. Restriction of use is not currently recommended, even in women at high risk of HIV infection; however, consistent co-use of condoms is advised.

- For those seeking emergency contraception a copper intrauterine device is first line. If an oral method is preferred, doubling the dose of levonorgestrel (3 mg) is recommended for women taking ART.
- Women who have HIV-negative partners (i.e. discordant couples) should also be advised of the availability of post-exposure prophylaxis following sexual exposure (PEPSE).

3.4 Women with inflammatory bowel disease (IBD)

IBD, including ulcerative colitis and Crohn's disease, can present at any age, though it frequently presents between the ages of 10 and 40 years. The appropriateness of a means of contraception in women with IBD depends on a number of factors:
- the impact of the IBD on an individual's digestive tract
- the impact of IBD-associated conditions such as VTE and osteoporosis
- the medications used in IBD management such as corticosteroids, immunosuppressants, 5-aminosalicylic acid drugs and anti-tumour necrosis factor alpha agents.

There is no evidence of a causal relationship between exacerbations of IBD and combined contraceptive use.
- The efficacy of oral contraceptives is not reduced in women with large bowel disease. However, it may be reduced in women with small bowel disease and malabsorption.
- Rectal preparations for IBD, such as oil- or Witepsol-based products, may reduce the efficacy of barrier methods if the product spreads to genital skin, therefore checking the constituents is recommended before prescribing.
- Laparoscopic sterilization is not a recommended method of contraception for women with IBD who have had previous surgery. In these circumstances a LARC, hysteroscopic sterilization or vasectomy present a more appropriate alternative.

3.4.1 Pregnancy and IBD

- Pregnancy is contraindicated in women taking some of the medication used to manage IBD, such as methotrexate due to teratogenicity (irrespective of which partner is using this medication), or infliximab. Therefore, effective contraception is required for the duration of use and often for several months after completion of treatment. The summary of product characteristics for the individual medications can be reviewed for information and advice regarding pregnancy and breast-feeding.
- Effective contraception also enables individuals with IBD to optimize their management prior to conception and plan a pregnancy when their disease is well-controlled.

3.5 Women with cardiovascular disease

- For young women with cardiovascular disease, the provision of contraception and sexual health advice should ideally occur as part of transitional care from paediatric to adult services. Discussions should cover sexual health and risks associated with pregnancy, not just which methods of contraception are suitable for the young person.

- Involving the young woman and all members of the healthcare team, including the individual's cardiologist, ensures both medical and personal acceptability of the contraceptive method.
- CHCs are associated with an increased risk of VTE and are often contraindicated in women with cardiovascular disease.
- Prophylactic antibiotics are not required for the insertion of intrauterine contraceptives (IUCs) in women at risk of infective endocarditis. More complex individual cases, such as those with a past history of endocarditis or prosthetic heart valve, should be discussed with the woman's cardiologist.
- In those at increased risk from vasovagal reactions, IUC fitting should occur within a hospital setting, with appropriate resuscitation support at hand.
- The use of anticoagulant therapy need not restrict the provision of progestogen-only implants, injectables or IUCs.
- A desogestrel-containing progestogen-only contraceptive pill is a useful interim method (except for women using liver enzyme inducers) to prevent pregnancy while obtaining further information and clarification from the woman's cardiologist.

3.6 Drug interactions

- Prior to the provision of contraception it is important to ask about current medication, including over-the-counter and herbal remedies and ascertain if they interact with the chosen method.
- Likewise, before new medication is taken women are advised to discuss their current contraception use in order to avoid potential drug interactions.
- Liver enzyme inducing drugs reduce the bioavailability of oestrogen and progestogen and so potentially reduce the contraceptive efficacy of several methods of contraception.
- Progestogen-only injectables, the intrauterine system (IUS) and the intrauterine device (IUD) are unaffected by liver enzyme inducing drugs.
- It is advisable for women to use additional barrier methods or change to an injectable or IUC when liver enzyme inducing medications are commenced (see *Table 3.1* for common liver enzyme inducing drugs).

Table 3.1. Liver enzyme inducing drugs

Drug category	Medication	
Antibiotic	Rifabutin Rifampicin	
Antiepileptic	Carbamazepine Eslicarbazepine Phenytoin	Primidone Rifinamide Topiramate (only in daily doses of >200 mg)
Antiretroviral	Efavirenz Nevirapine	Ritonavir Ritonavir-boosted medications
Herbal	St John's wort	
Other	Aprepitant Bosentan	

- Some women will only use enzyme inducing medications on a short-term basis and may wish to remain on their current combined hormonal method, progestogen-only pill or implant. The addition of a barrier method for the duration of the treatment and for 28 days after stopping the drug is recommended as an alternative to a change in method.
  - If a CHC is to be continued, prescribe a COC with a minimum of 30 mcg ethinylestradiol or a patch or vaginal ring. Advocate an extended cycle regimen or tricycling (taking 3 packets back to back) and reduce the hormone-free interval to 4 days PLUS use a barrier method.
  - Alternatively, increase ethinylestradiol to at least 50 mcg (taking a 20 and 30 mcg COC) using the extended cycle regimen or tricycling with a 4 day hormone-free interval. Using two vaginal rings or two patches is not recommended. This is also not advised for those taking rifampicin or rifabutin.
  - The dose of ethinylestradiol can be increased up to 70 mcg (two 35 mcg COCs daily) if breakthrough bleeding occurs when taking the liver enzyme inducing medication, providing other causes of bleeding have been excluded (see *Chapter 4*).
- If emergency contraception is required, a copper IUD is first line due to the potential interaction between oral emergency contraception and liver enzyme inducing drugs. If an IUD is declined or unsuitable a 3 mg dose (double dose) of oral levonorgestrel as soon as possible within 120 hours of unprotected sex can be used. This use is outside the product licence.
- Ulipristal acetate (emergency contraception) is not advised for women currently using, or who have used enzyme inducing drugs in the last 28 days.
- There is no need to use additional contraception during or after a course of non-enzyme inducing antibiotics.
- CHC and lamotrigine monotherapy are not recommended due to the risk of reduced seizure control whilst on CHC and potential toxicity during the CHC-free interval. All other methods are suitable.
- A useful drug interactions checker is provided by Medscape at http://reference.medscape.com/drug-interactionchecker

3.7 Women with learning disabilities

- Learning disabilities are a spectrum of disorders wherein an individual has a significantly reduced ability to understand new or complex information and may be unable to live independently. Women with learning disabilities should be supported to make their own decisions about contraception. A person with a learning disability may still be competent to make an informed choice regarding a method of contraception and be able to use any method reliably, including an oral method. Discussion of available options is based on medical assessment and the acceptability of a method to a given individual, not their learning disability.

3.7.1 Consent and capacity

- To be deemed competent women must demonstrate an ability to understand and retain the information provided, weigh up the risks and benefits and express their wishes as set out in the Mental Capacity Act 2005 for England and

Wales. The Act applies to all individuals aged 16 years and over. Under the Act a person is presumed to be competent unless they have demonstrated otherwise. Competence is decision-specific and cannot be generalized to all medical situations.

- When a woman with a learning disability is unable to understand and take responsibility for her decisions about contraception, a meeting between carers and other involved parties is advised. This discussion aims to establish a care plan, address issues around the woman's contraceptive need but also consider the individual's wishes too. Any decision made is in the best interests of the individual and generally the least restrictive option. No one individual can consent for another.
- If a woman has no-one (other than paid carers) to support and represent her, or when a serious medical treatment such as sterilization or abortion is proposed, an Independent Mental Capacity Advocate (IMCA) is appointed. Their role is to support an individual to ensure that they can participate in decision making, to determine their wishes, beliefs and values, and to discuss alternative options. Those involved in the care of an individual with an IMCA are obliged to take into consideration submissions made by the IMCA.
- When making decisions regarding contraception for an individual with learning disabilities the best interests of that person are paramount rather than the most convenient option for those involved in supporting/caring for that individual. Importantly, carers cannot give consent for another individual.
- The Court of Protection was established under the Mental Capacity Act and its role is to protect those who lack capacity and make rulings on difficult decisions regarding their care. An application may be made to the Court of Protection by a family member, hospital trust or local authority. The decision making process involves the individual who lacks capacity. A 'litigation friend' is appointed to provide legal instruction; this may be a friend, relative or solicitor. If no-one is available, an official solicitor is appointed to act as a litigation friend during the Court of Protection process.

3.8 Women with physical disabilities

- It is important to consider the impact of a physical disability on an individual's mobility when discussing contraceptive options.
- For women with very limited mobility it is wise to review their baseline risk of VTE and the impact of the additional risk associated with oestrogen-containing methods of contraception before prescribing.
- For women with limited mobility or those with a medical condition which may affect bone mineral density, careful consideration of the risks and benefits is advisable before prescribing progestogen-only injectable contraceptives (see *Section 6.6*).
- For those with limited dexterity, for example, due to arthritis, consideration should be given to the administration of contraceptive methods to ensure that their disability does not unduly limit their choice of contraception. Dexterity may limit the ability of an individual to utilize oral contraceptives or patches or vaginal rings.

3.9 Women with sensory disabilities

3.9.1 Visual impairment

- Research indicates that young adults with visual impairments have similar rates of sexual experiences as their sighted counterparts; however, their experience typically occurs 2–3 years later, highlighting the importance of considering their sexual health needs.
- The provision of information in large print, Braille or as a recording is important for clients with visual impairments.
- For visually impaired women wishing to use a COC or a POP, the pharmacy or family members may need to include the contraceptive in a 'dosette box'. This will help compliance and ensure this method of contraception is an option for visually impaired women because Braille packaging is not generally available.

3.9.2 Hearing impairment

- For women with hearing impairments who lip read, face to face consultation with slow, clear articulation, avoiding over-exaggerated facial expression, can be adequate to ensure an effective consultation. Individuals with a strongly accented voice may find it more difficult to undertake the consultation because accents can make lip reading more difficult.
- The provision of an interpreter for deaf clients may be required, depending on clinician or client request, with care taken to ensure privacy but also to ensure the woman has a 'voice' during intimate examinations.

3.10 Women who do not speak English

- For clients who do not have English as a first language the provision of an interpreter may be needed.
- The interpreter should not be a family member, but an independent individual who acts purely as a channel for communication. The interpreter may be physically present at the time of the consultation or participate via telephone.
- For intimate examinations, it is generally recommended that an interpreter is present within the consultation room.

EXAMPLE

A 24 year old woman with learning disabilities attends with her mum who is requesting a sterilization for her daughter.

What should you do?

1. Discuss the reasons behind the request.
2. Ascertain the young woman's wishes through an IMCA if necessary.
3. Consider less permanent options.
4. Refer to the Court of Protection if a decision cannot be reached.

References

Fakoya, A. (2007) *UK guidelines for the management of sexual and reproductive health (SRH) of people living with HIV infection.* BASHH and BHIVA.
[available at www.bashh.org – accessed April 2016]

FSRH (2009) *Sexual and Reproductive Health for Individuals with Inflammatory Bowel Disease.* Clinical Effectiveness Unit.
[www.fsrh.org/documents/ceuguidanceibd09/ – accessed June 2016]

FSRH (2010) *Contraception for Women Aged Over 40.* Clinical Effectiveness Unit.
[www.fsrh.org/documents/cec-ceu-guidance-womenover40-jul-2010/ – accessed June 2016]

FSRH (2010) *Contraceptive Choices for Young People.* Clinical Effectiveness Unit.
[www.fsrh.org/documents/cec-ceu-guidance-young-people-mar-2010/ – accessed June 2016]

FSRH (2012) *Drug Interactions with Hormonal Contraception.* Clinical Effectiveness Unit.
[www.fsrh.org/documents/ceu-guidance-drug-interactions-with-hormonal-contraception-jan/ – accessed June 2016]

FSRH (2014) *Contraceptive Choices for Women with Cardiac Disease.* Clinical Effectiveness Unit.
[www.fsrh.org/documents/ceu-guidance-contraceptive-choices-for-women-with-cardiac/ – accessed June 2016]

Mental Capacity Act (2005)
[www.legislation.gov.uk/ukpga/2005/9/contents – accessed April 2016]

Ralph, L.J. *et al.* (2015) Hormonal contraceptive use and women's risk of HIV acquisition: a meta-analysis of observational studies. *Lancet Infectious Diseases,* **15(2):** 181–189.
[http://dx.doi.org/10.1016/S1473-3099(14)71052-7 – accessed April 2016]

Chapter 4

Combined hormonal contraception

Approximately 3 million UK women use the combined oral contraceptive (COC).

Combined hormonal contraceptives (CHCs) contain both oestrogen and progestogen. There are three routes of administration: oral (pill), transdermal (combined transdermal patch, CTP) and vaginal (combined vaginal ring, CVR).

In addition to its contraceptive indication, CHC is prescribed to help manage menstrual symptoms including dysmenorrhoea, premenstrual syndrome, heavy menstrual bleeding and acne. Only one product (Qlaira) has a licence for the treatment of heavy menstrual bleeding in those who desire contraception. Prescribing solely to treat a non-contraceptive benefit is seen as an off-licence indication.

4.1 Potential users

4.1.1 Most appropriate users

- CHCs can be used from menarche to the age of 50 years providing there are no contraindicating risk factors or medical conditions. For those over 50, healthcare professionals can use their clinical judgement if the benefits are thought to outweigh the potential risks.
- CHCs are an ideal choice for women who wish to have a regular bleed or to control when they have a withdrawal bleed.
- Individuals should choose whether they wish to use oral, transdermal or vaginal CHCs.

4.1.2 Not suitable for the following users

CHCs are not suitable for the following women (for more information see UKMEC in *Appendix*):
- those suffering from migraine with aura

- those with current or recent breast cancer
- those breast-feeding and less than 6 weeks post-partum
- those less than 3 weeks post-partum or less than 6 weeks post-partum with other risk factors for VTE
- those with a BMI over 35 kg/m^2
- those with hypertension
- those over 35 years of age who currently smoke, including those who smoke electronic cigarettes, as the risk associated with electronic cigarette smoking has not yet been established
- those with multiple risk factors for arterial cardiovascular disease
- those with current or past VTE, or with VTE in a first-degree relative under the age of 45, or a known thrombogenic mutation
- those with known genetic mutation associated with breast cancer
- those with diabetes with retinopathy, nephropathy, neuropathy or other vascular disease
- prolonged immobility including following surgery
- those with acute or flare of viral hepatitis
- those with cirrhosis or liver tumours
- those with a current or history of ischaemic heart disease
- those with a current or history of stroke
- those with positive antiphospholipid antibodies.

4.2 Available CHC in the UK

CHCs available in the UK are detailed in *Table 4.1*, along with associated costs and formulations.

Table 4.1. CHCs available in the UK

Type of preparation	Trade name	Oestrogen and progestogen	Cost for 3 cycles
Monophasic low strength, 21 days	Gedarel 20/150 Mercilon	Ethinylestradiol 20 mcg and desogestrel 150 mcg	£5.98 £8.44
	Femodette Millinette 20/75 Sunya 20/75	Ethinylestradiol 20 mcg and gestodene 75 mcg	£8.85 £6.37 £6.62
	Loestrin 20	Ethinylestradiol 20 mcg and norethisterone acetate 1 mg	£2.70
Monophasic standard strength, 21 days	Gedarel 30/150 Marvelon	Ethinylestradiol 30 mcg and desogestrel 150 mcg	£4.93 £7.10
	Yasmin Lucette	Ethinylestradiol 30 mcg and drospirenone 3 mg	£14.70 £9.35
	Femodene Katya 30/75 Millinette 30/75	Ethinylestradiol 30 mcg and gestodene 75 mcg	£6.73 £5.03 £4.85

Type of preparation	Trade name	Oestrogen and progestogen			Cost for 3 cycles
Monophasic standard strength, 21 days (*cont.*)	Levest Microgynon 30 Ovranette Rigevidon	Ethinylestradiol 30 mcg and levonorgestrel 150 mcg			£1.80 £2.82 £2.20 £1.89
	Loestrin 30	Ethinylestradiol 30 mcg and norethisterone acetate 1.5 mg			£3.90
	Cilest Cilique	Ethinylestradiol 35 mcg and norgestimate 250 mcg Ethinylestradiol 35 mcg and norgestimate 250 mcg			£7.16 £4.65
	Brevinor Ovysmen	Ethinylestradiol 35 mcg and norethisterone 500 mcg			£1.99 £1.89
	Norimin	Ethinylestradiol 35 mcg and norethisterone 1 mg			£2.28
	Norinyl-1	Mestranol 50 mcg and norethisterone 1 mg			£2.19
Monophasic standard strength, every day 21 active and 7 inactive	Femodene ED	Ethinylestradiol 30 mcg and gestodene 75 mcg			£7.10
	Microgynon 30 ED	Ethinylestradiol 30 mcg and levonorgestrel 150 mcg			£2.99
Monophasic every day, 24 active and 4 inactive	Zoely	Oestradiol (as hemihydrate) 1.5 mg and nomegestrol acetate 2.5 mg			£19.80
	Daylette Eloine	Ethinylestradiol 20 mcg and drospirenone 3 mg			£10.50 £14.70
Phasic standard strength, 21 days	Triadene	Ethinylestradiol 30 mcg Ethinylestradiol 40 mcg Ethinylestradiol 30 mcg	Gestodene 50 mcg Gestodene 70 mcg Gestodene 100 mcg	6 5 10	£10.40
	Logynon TriRegol	Ethinylestradiol 30 mcg Ethinylestradiol 30 mcg Ethinylestradiol 30 mcg	Levonorgestrel 50 mcg Levonorgestrel 75 mcg Levonorgestrel 125 mcg	6 5 10	£3.82 £2.87
	BiNovum	Ethinylestradiol 35 mcg Ethinylestradiol 35 mcg	Norethisterone 0.5 mg Norethisterone 1 mg	7 14	£2.49
	Synphase	Ethinylestradiol 35 mcg Ethinylestradiol 35 mcg Ethinylestradiol 35 mcg	Norethisterone 0.5 mg Norethisterone 1 mg Norethisterone 0.5 mg	7 9 5	1-cycle pack = £1.20
	TriNovum	Ethinylestradiol 35 mcg Ethinylestradiol 35 mcg Ethinylestradiol 35 mcg	Norethisterone 0.5 mg Norethisterone 0.75 mg Norethisterone 1 mg	7 7 7	£3.46
Phasic standard strength every day, 21 active and 7 inactive	Logynon ED	Ethinylestradiol 30 mcg Ethinylestradiol 30 mcg Ethinylestradiol 30 mcg	Levonorgestrel 50 mcg Levonorgestrel 75 mcg Levonorgestrel 125 mcg	6 5 10	£4.00

Type of preparation	Trade name	Oestrogen and progestogen			Cost for 3 cycles
Phasic every day, 26 active and 2 inactive	Qlaira	Oestradiol valerate 3 mg	Dienogest 2 mg	2	£25.18
		Oestradiol valerate 2 mg	Dienogest 2 mg	5	
		Oestradiol valerate 2 mg	Dienogest 3 mg	17	
		Oestradiol valerate 1 mg	Dienogest 3 mg	2	
Patch	Evra	Ethinylestradiol approx. 33.9 mcg/24 hours			£19.51
		Norelgestromin approx. 203 mcg/24 hours			
Ring	NuvaRing	Ethinylestradiol approx. 15 mcg/24 hours			£29.70
		Etonogestrel approx. 120 mcg/24 hours			

Data from *British National Formulary* 2015.

4.3 Mechanism of action

- The main mode of action is prevention of ovulation through negative feedback on the pituitary gland, inhibiting the release of luteinizing hormone (LH) and follicle-stimulating hormone (FSH). In formulations with 21 days of active hormone, the first 7 days of CHC use results in ovulation inhibition and the next 14 days maintains anovulation.
- Cervical mucus is altered which inhibits penetration of spermatozoa.
- Endometrial growth is suppressed, reducing the likelihood of blastocyst implantation.

4.4 Efficacy of CHC

If used consistently and correctly the failure rate for CHC is 0.3% (in the first year of use 3 in 1000 women would become pregnant) but this increases to 9% with typical use.

4.5 Pros and cons of CHC

4.5.1 Advantages

- Effective, reversible, convenient.
- Under user's control and unrelated to sexual intercourse.
- Provides regular, predictable withdrawal bleeds.
- Reduces menstrual loss by at least 40% – recommended by NICE (CG44, 2007) for the treatment of heavy menstrual bleeding.
- Decreases dysmenorrhoea and relieves ovulation pain.
- Reduces acne.
- May improve premenstrual symptoms.
- Protects against ectopic pregnancy because it inhibits ovulation.
- Reduces incidence of benign breast disease.

- Reduces the risk of ovarian cancer. A recent meta-analysis determined a significant duration–response relationship, with a reduction in the incidence of ovarian cancer of more than 50% among women using the CHC for 10 years or more (Havrilesky, 2006). This protection continues for at least 20 years after discontinuation.
- Reduction in functional ovarian cysts and fibroid formation.
- Reduces risk of endometrial cancer by at least 50%. This protection increases with duration of use and continues for at least 15 years after CHC is discontinued.
- Incidence of bowel cancer is reduced by 20%. However, longer duration of use does not appear to confer greater reduction in risk.
- CHC use reduces the incidence of endometriosis and improves the symptoms associated with this condition.
- Helps to protect against pelvic inflammatory disease.
- Menopausal symptoms may be reduced. Extended use or a reduced pill-free interval may further improve symptom control.

4.5.2 Disadvantages

- These methods must be used correctly and consistently to be effective.
- Drug interactions reduce efficacy.
- Patches cause local skin reaction in up to 20% of users.
- Vaginal ring causes 'vaginitis' in 5–14% of women.
- CHC does not provide protection against STIs.
- There may be an increased risk of breast cancer. A frequently quoted re-analysis study (Collaborative Group on Hormonal Factors in Breast Cancer, 1996) suggested a 24% increased risk of developing breast cancer above background in CHC users. It suggested risk increases after commencing CHC, returning to background level 10 years after stopping. However, there was no effect of dose or duration on breast cancer incidence. A number of recent studies have found no associated risk with the low dose CHC formulations currently prescribed.
- After 5 years of use, these methods may be associated with an increase in the incidence of cervical intraepithelial neoplasia (CIN) and cancer of the cervix. The combined hormonal components appear to be a co-factor leading to persistence or repeated replication of oncogenic human papilloma virus. Those taking CHC should be advised to have regular cervical screening as indicated by the NHS cervical screening programme (NHSCSP). Women who have previously been treated for CIN may choose to take a CHC because the benefits outweigh the potential risks. They should be advised to continue cervical screening as indicated by the NHSCSP.
- There may be a very small increased risk of MI in CHC users. This risk is increased in women who smoke (up to 20-fold increased risk) and in those with hypertension.
- There is a two-fold increased risk of ischaemic stroke in CHC users. This corresponds to a small absolute risk because the incidence of ischaemic stroke in women under 35 is 3 per 100 000 each year. There is no increased risk of haemorrhagic stroke associated with CHC use.
- *Table 4.2* details the risk of VTE associated with CHC use.

Table 4.2. Risk of developing a VTE in a year

Women **not using** a combined hormonal pill/patch/ring and who are not pregnant	About 2 out of 10 000 women
Women who are pregnant or in the immediate post-partum period	About 29 out of 10 000 women
Women using a CHC containing **levonorgestrel, norethisterone or norgestimate**	About 5–7 out of 10 000 women
Women using a CHC containing **etonogestrel or norelgestromin**	About 6–12 out of 10 000 women
Women using a CHC containing **drospirenone, gestodene or desogestrel**	About 9–12 out of 10 000 women
Women using a CHC containing **dienogest or nomegestrol acetate**	Not yet known

Data from MHRA (2014).

4.6 Using the CHC

Prior to starting the CHC, documentation of blood pressure and BMI is recommended, along with a relevant medical history to determine any contraindications (see *Chapters 1 and 2*). Before being prescribed CHC, women need to be made aware of the symptoms and risks of VTE and other indications to immediately stop taking CHCs (see *Section 4.6.8*).

4.6.1 Conventional use

- For most preparations the CHC is taken daily for 21 days followed by a 7 day pill-free or placebo pill interval, during which time a withdrawal bleed will occur. Apps are available to help users remember to take their pills.
- The CTP is changed every 7 days for 3 weeks followed by a patch-free week.
- The CVR is inserted into the vagina and remains in place for 3 weeks followed by a ring-free week.
- All of the methods have similar efficacy, but the CTP and CVR are advantageous for women who cannot remember a daily pill or who have gastrointestinal problems affecting pill absorption.
- When commencing CHC, the method prescribed should suit the majority of women, have a proven safety record and be inexpensive. A CHC containing 30 mcg ethinylestradiol and levonorgestrel fulfils these criteria and is therefore a good first choice.
- The CHCs containing oestradiol and nomegestrol acetate (including four placebo tablets in each 28 day cycle) or containing oestradiol valerate and dienogest (including two placebo tablets in each 28 day cycle) are taken daily. The latter has an oestrogenic step-down and progestogenic step-up dosing regimen, reducing the incidence of breakthrough bleeding associated with oestradiol-containing pills. Both of these pills are associated with a shorter withdrawal bleed (3–4 days for the former and 4 days for the latter) compared to other CHCs (typically 5 days) and a higher likelihood of missing a withdrawal bleed (30% for oestradiol and nomegestrol compared to 5% with drospirenone-containing CHCs, and 19.4% for oestradiol valerate and dienogest). A pregnancy test is advised if two withdrawal bleeds are missed.

4.6.2 Extended or flexible use (off licence)

- There is no medical reason to have a monthly withdrawal bleed.
- Extended use can be recommended for CHC, CTP and CVR users; back to back use for 3 cycles, i.e. 3 packets of pills, 9 patches or 3 rings. This is followed by a 7 day or 4 day interval, after which the method is recommenced.
- Alternatively, the chosen CHC method can be used flexibly with continuous use for at least 21 days. Then if troublesome breakthrough bleeding occurs for 3–4 days the CHC can be stopped for an interval of 4 or 7 days. It is then recommenced for at least a further 21 days before another break is made. If no breakthrough bleeding occurs the CHC can be used continuously with no break.

4.6.3 Vomiting and severe diarrhoea

- Efficacy of CHCs can be affected by vomiting and severe diarrhoea.
- If vomiting occurs within 2 hours of taking the CHC, another pill should be taken and no further action is needed.
- If the vomiting continues or severe diarrhoea occurs it is advisable to follow the missed pills advice (see *Section 4.6.6*).

4.6.4 Drug interactions

- Non-enzyme inducing antibiotics such as amoxycillin do not affect the efficacy of CHCs.
- Liver enzyme inducing drugs such as carbamazepine, phenytoin and topiramate (more than 200 mg per day) increase the metabolism of both oestrogen and progestogen, thereby reducing the contraceptive efficacy of CHC (see *Chapter 2*).
- Lamotrigine monotherapy with CHC use may result in a reduction in serum levels of lamotrigine. It could result in an increased seizure frequency during CHC use and toxicity risk during the CHC-free interval. Therefore concomitant use is not recommended.

4.6.5 Starting regimens

These are described in *Table 4.3* below.

4.6.6 Advice about missed or late CHC

- A missed pill is one which is taken more than 24 hours after the pill was due but less than 48 hours late (48–72 hours since the last pill was taken).
- If one pill is missed, it should be taken as soon as it is remembered and the rest of the pack should be continued. No further action is generally required.

Table 4.3. Starting regimens for CHCs

Circumstances	Start when?	Extra precautions for seven days? (Nine days for oestradiol valerate and dienogest-containing CHC)
Quick starting	At any time if it is reasonably certain that the woman is not pregnant	Yes
Menstruating	Up to and including day 5	No
	After day 5 of the cycle	Yes
Amenorrhoeic	Any time if it is reasonably certain that the patient is not pregnant	Yes
Post-abortion or miscarriage	Within 5 days	No
	After 5 days	Yes
Post-partum (a) not breast-feeding	Day 21 postpartum	No
	From day 22 onwards	Yes
(b) breast-feeding	If >6 weeks treat like other menstruating or amenorrhoeic women	Yes
Switching from other hormonal methods (other than IUS)	Immediate start	No
	If previous method was DMPA, switch when next injection is due	No
Switching from a non-hormonal method (other than IUD)	Up to and including day 5	No
	After day 5	Yes
Switching from an IUD or IUS	Start up to and including day 5 of cycle. IUD/IUS can be removed at the same time	No
	CHC can be started at any other time, if it is reasonably certain she is not pregnant:	
	– if she has been sexually active	Start CHC and then remove IUD/IUS at the next period or after 7 days
	– if she has not been sexually active	Start CHC and then remove IUD/IUS after 7 days or at the next period. Alternatively, start CHC, remove IUD/IUS and advise additional contraception for 7 days
	– if she is amenorrhoeic or has irregular bleeds	Start CHC; if unprotected sex in the preceding 7 days advise IUD/IUS removal 7 days after pill start

- If two or more pills are missed (i.e. more than 72 hours since last pill was taken or more than 48 hours late in restarting pill after pill-free interval) see *Table 4.4* for advice.

Table 4.4. Missed pills advice

Pills missed	Guidance
If two or more pills are missed in the first week or more than 48 hours late restarting CHC	• Take most recent missed pill • Continue with the rest of the pack and use condoms or abstain for the next 7 days • If sexual intercourse occurred in the preceding 7 days, emergency contraception may be needed (see *Chapter 13*)
Two or more missed pills and more than 7 pills left in the packet	• Take the most recent missed pill even if this means taking 2 pills on one day • Continue with the rest of the pack and use condoms or abstain for the next 7 days • Finish packet and have the pill-free interval as usual
Two or more missed pills and less than 7 pills left in the packet	• Take the most recent missed pill even if this means taking 2 pills on one day • Continue with the rest of the pack and use condoms or abstain for the next 7 days • Omit the pill-free interval, finish the active tablets in the current packet and immediately start a new packet; do not take any of the inactive or placebo tablets

If a CHC containing oestradiol and nomegestrol is taken less than 12 hours late there is no reduction in contraceptive efficacy. If the pill is taken more than 12 hours late see *Table 4.5* for missed pills advice.

Table 4.5. Missed pills advice – oestradiol- and nomegestrol-containing CHCs

When pills missed	Guidance
Day 1–7	• Take the pill when it is remembered, even if it means taking 2 tablets at the same time • Use barrier methods for next 7 days; consider EC
Day 8–17	• 1 tablet missed, take it when remembered, no condoms needed unless more pills have been missed • >1 tablet missed, use condoms for next 7 days
Day 18–24	Option 1: skip placebo pills, no additional need for condom use providing no missed pills in the preceding 7 days; may get some menstrual spotting
	Option 2: stop taking active pills and immediately take the 4 placebo tablets and then start next pack

If one CHC pill containing oestradiol valerate and dienogest is taken more than 12 hours late the missed pills advice in *Table 4.6* is recommended.

Table 4.6. Missed pills advice – oestradiol valerate- and dienogest-containing CHCs

When pills missed	Guidance
Day 1–17	Take the missed pill as soon as possible, even if it means taking 2 pills at the same time Continue taking pills according normal use Use barrier method for 9 days
Day 18–24	Discard remaining pills, start new packet and take normally Use barrier method for 9 days
Day 25–26	Take the missed pill as soon as possible, even if it means taking 2 pills at the same time No barrier method needed
Day 27–28	Discard missed pill and continue taking the packet as normal; no barrier method needed

4.6.7 Advice regarding incorrect use of the CTP and CVR

- If the patch- or ring-free interval is extended by less than 48 hours, no additional contraception is required.
- If the patch- or ring-free interval is extended by more than 48 hours, additional contraception or abstinence from sexual intercourse is needed for 7 days. There may be a need for emergency contraception if sexual intercourse occurred in the patch- or ring-free interval (see *Chapter 13*).
- If the CTP or CVR is detached or removed for less than 48 hours, no additional contraception is required, providing that the method has been correctly used for the preceding 7 days. If the CTP or CVR is detached or removed for more than 48 hours, additional contraception is needed for the next 7 days; if this occurs in week one and unprotected sexual intercourse occurred in the patch- or ring-free interval, emergency contraception may be needed (see *Chapter 13*).
- If the CTP remains in place for 9 days or fewer, or the CVR remains *in situ* for 4 weeks or fewer, no additional contraception is needed and the patch- or ring-free interval can be taken. However, if the CTP is in place for more than 9 days or the CVR is in place for more than 5 weeks, additional contraception or abstinence is needed for 7 days. The patch- or ring-free interval should be missed and a new cycle commenced. If the CVR has been in place for more than 4 weeks but less than 5 weeks, efficacy can be maintained by missing the ring-free interval and inserting a new CVR.

4.6.8 When to stop using CHC immediately

If any of the following occur the CHC should be stopped immediately:
- sudden severe chest pain
- breathlessness
- haemoptysis
- unexplained swelling or severe pain in calf of one leg
- weakness, numbness or severe pins and needles in an arm or leg
- severe stomach pain

- bad fainting attack or collapse
- unusual severe, prolonged headaches or new migraine
- sudden partial or complete loss of vision or sudden disturbance of hearing or other perceptual disorders or dysphasia
- first unexplained epileptic seizure or weakness, motor disturbances, very marked numbness suddenly affecting one side or one part of body
- hepatitis, jaundice, liver enlargement
- blood pressure above 160 mmHg systolic or 95 mmHg diastolic
- detection of a risk factor which contraindicates treatment.

4.6.9 Surgery and immobility

- VTE risk in CHC users is further increased with prolonged immobility and following major surgery.
- Women should discuss discontinuing the CHC with their surgeon.
- It is normally advised that CHC should be stopped 4 weeks prior to major elective surgery, surgery to the lower limbs, and surgery which will result in prolonged immobility but not for minor or short duration surgery.
- Alternative contraceptive options should be discussed and commenced to avoid unplanned pregnancy. All progestogen-only methods are suitable in this situation.
- The CHC can be recommenced at least 2 weeks after full mobilization.

4.7 Routine follow-up

- Initially a 3 month supply should be given. This is followed by a review to assess any problems and check blood pressure.
- Once stable on a CHC, a year's supply can be issued (with the exception of the CVR which will need to be prescribed every 3 months). An annual review is undertaken to assess the recent medical and family history along with current medication. Blood pressure and BMI are also checked.
- CHCs can be used during the peri-menopause in non-smoking women with no other contraindications and may reduce menopausal symptoms.
- CHCs can be continued until the age of 50 after which an alternative method is advised. This should be continued until the age of 55 years by which time 98% of women will be at least 1 year past their last menstrual period (see *Chapter 2*).

4.8 Return to fertility

- There is no delay in return to fertility.
- The earliest estimated date of ovulation following missed combined pills or cessation of CHC is 10 days. Typically, ovulation occurs within 1 month of stopping CHC use.
- Conception rate is 72–94% within 12 months of ceasing CHC use.

4.9 Managing side-effects

Unscheduled bleeding is one of the most common side-effects, reported by approximately 20% of CHC users. This generally resolves over the first 3 months of use.

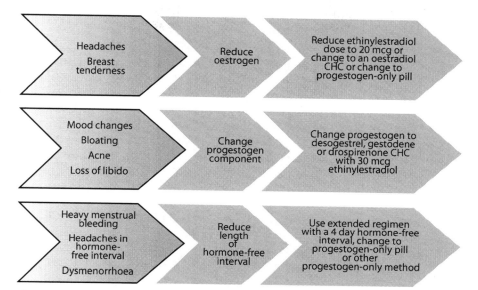

Figure 4.1. Side-effect management options.

Hormonally-associated side-effects include:

- **Nausea** – taking the pill at night may improve symptoms; alternatively a CVR or CTP could also be tried.
- **Breast tenderness** – a support bra or evening primrose oil for cyclical pain may be tried prior to a change in CHC.
- **Chloasma** (skin discolouration) – the use of skin block is recommended in conjunction with stopping the CHC and changing to POP, although it may continue with POP.
- **Acne** – lifestyle, diet and skin care advice are an initial management approach. If acne continues, change progestogen to desogestrel, gestodene or drospirenone CHC with 30 mcg ethinylestradiol. If it continues after 3 months add in topical or systemic treatment. If acne fails to improve after 6 months, change to cyproterone acetate and 35 mcg ethinylestradiol.
- **Hirsutism** – change to a drospirenone with 30 mcg ethinylestradiol CHC. If there is little response after 6 months, change to cyproterone acetate and 35 mcg ethinylestradiol.
- **Mood changes and loss of libido** – it is also important to explore relationship and personal issues.

CTP-specific side-effects include application site skin reaction in up to 20% of women. These reactions include irritation, redness, itch or rash. If they occur the patch should be removed and a new patch applied to another site. Skin reactions are an infrequent reason for discontinuation (2.6%).

CVR-specific side-effects include vaginitis (5.6%), vaginal discharge (4.8%) and awareness of the CVR during sexual intercourse (reported by 18% of women and 32% of partners). Foreign body sensation, coital problems and ring expulsion are less common, collectively affecting 4.4% of users.

4.10 Myths and misconceptions

- **CHCs should be stopped after 5 years of use** – there are no medical reasons to support women taking a break. Women who take a break and remain sexually active increase their risk of pregnancy. Taking a break from the CHC for 1 month or more then re-starting increases the risk of IMB and more significantly VTE. Additionally, the CHC has a duration-related protective effect for ovarian and endometrial cancer which supports continuation.
- **CHCs cause weight gain** – there is no evidence that CHCs cause weight gain. Weight fluctuates naturally due to changes in age or life circumstance; women tend to gain weight as they age.
- **CHCs reduce sexual desire and pleasure** – there is no evidence that CHCs affect a woman's sex drive.
- **CHCs cause acne** – although it is a common belief that CHCs cause acne, evidence suggests that CHCs may reduce acne lesions and those containing cyproterone acetate are licensed to treat severe acne.
- **CHCs must be stopped before air travel** – long-haul travel is a moderate risk factor for VTE. It is advisable that women keep well hydrated, avoid alcohol and undertake appropriate exercise to reduce immobility for flights lasting longer than 3 hours. The use of graduated compression stockings is not required for all women but may be indicated for women with additional risk factors.

EXAMPLE

A 27 year old attends for review to discuss irregular bleeding with her combined pill. She has taken it for 9 months.

What questions do you ask her? What are her contraceptive options if she wishes to continue to use a CHC?

1. Check compliance, pregnancy risk, malabsorption, drug interactions and undertake an STI risk assessment.
2. Check she has had a cervical screen within the last 3 years.
3. The CVR provides the best cycle control, with irregular bleeding occurring in just 2% of users compared to 39% in pill users. If she wishes to continue with a pill then a 30 mcg ethinylestradiol and 75 mcg gestodene, or 35 mcg ethinylestradiol and 250 mcg norgestimate would be good alternatives.
4. Alternatively she may wish to try a LARC.

References

British National Formulary, September 2014–March 2015.

Collaborative Group on Hormonal Factors in Breast Cancer (1996) Breast cancer and hormonal contraceptives: collaborative reanalysis of individual data on 53 297 women with breast cancer and 100 239 women without breast cancer from 54 epidemiological studies. *Lancet*, **347:** 1713–1727.

FSRH (2012) *Combined Hormonal Contraception.* Clinical Effectiveness Unit. [www.fsrh.org/documents/cec-ceu-guidance-chc-oct-2011/ – accessed June 2016]

Havrilesky, L.J. *et al.*(2013) Oral contraceptive pills as primary prevention for ovarian cancer: a systematic review and meta-analysis. *Obstetrics and Gynaecology,* 122 (1): 139–47.

MHRA (2014) Drug Safety Update: *Combined hormonal contraceptives and venous thromboembolism: review confirms risk is small.* [www.gov.uk/drug-safety-update/combined-hormonal-contraceptives-and-venous-thromboembolism-review-confirms-risk-is-small – accessed April 2016]

NICE (2007) CG44: *Heavy Menstrual Bleeding.* [www.nice.org.uk/guidance/cg44 – accessed April 2016]

Office for National Statistics (2009) Opinions Survey Report No. 41 *Contraception and Sexual Health,* 2008/09.

UKMEC (2016) *UK Medical Eligibility Criteria for Contraceptive Use* [www.fsrh.org/standards-and-guidance/uk-medical-eligibility-criteria-for-contraceptive-use/ – accessed June 2016]

Chapter 5
Progestogen-only pill

The progestogen-only pill (POP) is taken by about 6% of women aged 16–49 years in the UK, although it is less popular in other European countries.

5.1 Potential users

5.1.1 Most appropriate users

Almost all women who require contraception can take a POP (see UKMEC in *Appendix*).

5.1.2 Not suitable for the following users

The POP may not be effective in women taking liver enzyme inducing drugs and should be avoided in women who:
- have had a hormone-dependent tumour (e.g. breast cancer) in the last 5 years
- have severe decompensating cirrhosis or liver tumours
- are sensitive to any of the components of the POP
- are currently taking a POP and develop ischaemic heart or cerebrovascular disease.

5.2 Available POPs in the UK

These are listed in *Table 5.1*.

Table 5.1. POPs currently available in the UK

Trade name	Progestogen and dose	Cost
Micronor	Norethisterone, 350 mcg	3 × 28-tab pack = £1.80
Noriday		3 × 28-tab pack = £2.10
Norgeston	Levonorgestrel, 30 mcg	35-tab pack = £0.92
Cerazette Desogestrel	Desogestrel, 75 mcg	3 × 28-tab pack = £8.68 3 × 28-tab pack = £4.30

Data from *BNF*, 2015.

5.3 Mechanism of action

The mechanisms of action are illustrated in *Figure 5.1*.

- Ovulation may be suppressed in up to 60% of cycles in POPs containing levonorgestrel or norethisterone, but up to 97–99% in those containing desogestrel.
- All POPs alter the cervical mucus to reduce sperm penetration into the upper genital tract.
- POPs induce changes in the endometrium to prevent sperm survival and implantation of the blastocyst.
- Sperm motility and function is affected, preventing fertilization.

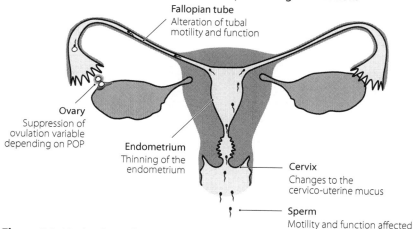

Figure 5.1. Mechanism of action for POPs.

5.4 Efficacy of POPs

The POP is very effective when taken consistently and correctly, with a 'perfect use' failure rate of less than 1%. However, the typical failure rate is 9% in the first year of use (see *Table 1.1*). The desogestrel POP is first line for most women as it is thought to be more effective than traditional POPs (as it usually inhibits ovulation and has a 12 rather than 3 hour safety window), but this has not been shown in any published study.

5.5 Pros and cons of POPs

5.5.1 Advantages

- Unrelated to sexual intercourse.
- Simple, convenient to use, and under the woman's control.
- Can be taken when breast-feeding.
- May help to reduce dysmenorrhoea and also severity of migraines.
- Ideal for women who suffer from oestrogenic side-effects when using CHC, e.g. breast tenderness, headaches including migraines, fluid retention, leg cramps or nausea.

- Suitable for women over 35 years who smoke.
- Can be used in overweight or obese women with no dose adjustment.
- Can be taken by those with medical illnesses where CHCs are contraindicated, e.g. women with hypertension, migraine with focal aura, or with a previous personal history of VTE.
- No evidence of an increased risk of cardiovascular disease, thromboembolism or stroke.
- Minimal alteration in carbohydrate and lipid metabolism, therefore a useful option for diabetics, even those with neuropathic or nephropathic complications.

5.5.2 Disadvantages

- Some women complain of nuisance side-effects such as breast tenderness, mood changes, headaches or acne.
- Possible risk of ectopic pregnancy in the event of POP failure.
- Can alter ovulation, thereby disrupting the menstrual bleeding pattern, with users reporting increased breakthrough bleeding, spotting and amenorrhoea.
- Functional ovarian cysts may develop in a small number of women; however, these tend to be transient and rarely require surgical intervention.

5.6 Using the POP

The POP is taken every day with no break. Following oral ingestion the effect on the cervical mucus reaches its peak within 2–3 hours then slowly wanes over the next 22 or so hours. POPs containing desogestrel differ from more traditional POPs because the main mode of action is to inhibit ovulation and so these POPs have a 12 hour rather than a 3 hour safety window. This means that women who normally take their traditional POP at 8 am have up to 11 am that day to take their pill. Those taking a desogestrel POP have until 8 pm that night (see advice on missed pills in *Section 5.6.2*).

The efficacy of the POP may be affected by vomiting or severe diarrhoea:
- If vomiting occurs within 2 hours of taking the POP, another pill is taken and no further action is required.
- If vomiting continues and/or she is 3 or more hours later than normal taking the pill (12 hours for a desogestrel POP), then the missed pill guidance should be followed.

The efficacy of the POP can be affected by concomitant use of a liver enzyme inducing drug, such as carbamazepine, phenobarbital, phenytoin, topiramate (200 mg or more a day), rifabutin, rifampicin, some antiretrovirals, ulipristal acetate, bosentan, and St John's wort.
- When these drugs are used short term, an additional method such as condoms should be used during the time of drug administration and for 4 weeks after stopping the medication.
- An alternative method such as an injectable or intrauterine contraceptive should be chosen if the liver enzyme inducing drug is to be used long term.

5.6.1 Starting regimens

Circumstances	Start when?	Extra precautions for 48 hours?
Quick start	At any time if it is reasonably certain that the woman is not pregnant	Yes
Menstruating	Up to and including day 5 of the cycle After day 5 of the cycle	No Yes
Amenorrhoea	At any time if it is reasonably certain that the woman is not pregnant	Yes
Post abortion or miscarriage	Within 5 days After 5 days	No Yes
Post-partum Breast-feeding or bottle feeding	Up to day 21 post-partum From day 22 onwards	No Yes
Switching from other hormonal methods (other than IUS)	Immediate start If previous method was DMPA, switch when next injection is due	No No
Switching from a non-hormonal method (other than IUD)	Up to and including day 5 After day 5	No Yes
Switching from an IUD or IUS	POP initiated at time of IUD/IUS removal (avoid unprotected sex or use condoms for 7 days before the removal of an IUD/IUS). POP started at least 2 days before the IUD/IUS is removed	Yes No

5.6.2 Advice about missed pills

- POPs are effective if taken consistently and correctly.
- If a norethisterone or levonorgestrel POP is forgotten for less than 3 hours from the normal administration time (the window is 12 hours for desogestrel POPs) the missed pill should be taken and the pack continued as normal. No additional cover such as condoms is required.
- If more than 3 hours has elapsed from the normal administration time (12 hours for desogestrel POP) then the last missed pill is taken, the pack continued as normal, but condoms should also be used as back-up contraception for the next 48 hours.
- If less than 3 hours has elapsed from the normal administration time (12 hours for desogestrel POP) and unprotected sex has occurred the missed pill should be taken, the POP continued and condoms used for the next 48 hours.
- If more than 3 hours has elapsed from the normal administration time (12 hours for desogestrel POP) and unprotected sex has occurred, emergency contraception should be considered (see *Chapter 13*).

5.7 Routine follow-up

After the first prescription for a POP women are given advice about when to return, normally in the next 3 months unless they have concerns. Once settled taking a POP they can be reviewed on an annual basis. POPs can be continued until the age of 55 when 98% of women are at least 1 year after their last natural period. For additional information see *Chapter 3*.

5.8 Return to fertility

There is no delay in return to fertility. Most women ovulate within 2–3 weeks of discontinuing POPs.

5.9 Managing side-effects

Non-specific symptoms such as headache, fatigue and mood change are common in the general population. Treatment-associated serious adverse reactions are very rare with POPs but an irregular bleeding pattern is common and some patients report possible progestogen-associated side-effects.

- In women taking POPs bleeding is unpredictable: 20% will have no periods, 40% irregular bleeding and 40% will have regular cycles. Those taking desogestrel rather than traditional POPs are more likely to have no or infrequent periods after 1 year of use.
- Encourage women to continue with the method for at least 3 months. In those with persistent troublesome bleeding, check compliance and drug interactions, exclude any STIs and pregnancy, examine the cervix and perform cervical cytology if due. Consider a change in POP or contraceptive method.
- Progestogen-associated side-effects may include acne, bloating, mood change and loss of libido. Again, encourage women to continue with the method for at least 3 months. If symptoms persist consider changing the POP to a different progestogen or consider a different method.
- There is no evidence that POPs increase or decrease weight.

5.10 Myths and misconceptions

- **POPs are not very effective in women weighing over 70 kg and these women need to take 2 POPs daily** – there is no evidence that POPs are less effective in overweight or obese women and so standard dosing regimens should be followed.
- **Women taking POPs and having amenorrhoea will have problems getting pregnant** – some women will not bleed while taking a POP. The endometrium is thin and atrophic. This is seen as an additional benefit, with many reporting reduced period pain too. On discontinuation of the POPs most women ovulate within the first 3 weeks and menstruate within the next 6 weeks. It has no effect on fertility.
- **Women with migraine with aura cannot take POPs** – this is not true. In fact many women with migraine with aura choose to take a POP for contraception because it may help reduce the intensity and frequency of the headache and aura.

> **EXAMPLE**
>
> **An 18 year old woman presents with painful, heavy periods; she also needs contraception. She would like to take the COC. History-taking establishes that her father experienced an unprovoked VTE at the age of 38 years, but there is no other family history of VTE. The family were genetically screened because her father was found to have factor V Leiden; only her sister was found to carry the gene for factor V Leiden.**
>
> *What do you advise?*
>
> 1. Using UKMEC this family history suggests that the risks of taking a COC outweigh any potential benefits (UKMEC 3), even though her thrombophilia screen was normal. This is because we can only look for known mutations and she may carry an increased VTE risk from an unknown alteration in genetic sequencing. This should be explained to the patient.
> 2. Alternatives with a lower risk for this woman would be a desogestrel POP, DMPA or a LNG-IUS.

References

British National Formulary, September 2014–March 2015.

FSRH (2010) *Contraception for Women Aged Over 40*. Clinical Effectiveness Unit. [www.fsrh.org/documents/cec-ceu-guidance-womenover40-jul-2010/ – accessed June 2016]

FSRH (2015) *Progestogen-only Pills*. Clinical Effectiveness Unit. [www.fsrh.org/documents/ceuguidanceprogestogenonlypills/ – accessed June 2016]

Office for National Statistics (2009) Opinions Survey Report No. 41 *Contraception and Sexual Health*, 2008/09.

UKMEC (2016) *UK Medical Eligibility Criteria for Contraceptive Use* [www.fsrh.org/standards-and-guidance/uk-medical-eligibility-criteria-for-contraceptive-use/ – accessed June 2016]

Chapter 6
Injectable contraception

Progestogen-only injectables have been available for over 40 years with a good safety record. About 3% of UK women aged between 16 and 49 years use a progestogen-only injectable as their method of contraception, with most users receiving depot medroxyprogesterone acetate (DMPA). Monthly combined injectables containing oestrogen and progestogens are available in Latin America but in few European countries. This chapter will discuss progestogen-only injectables, focusing on those containing medroxyprogesterone acetate.

6.1 Potential users

6.1.1 Most appropriate users

Injectable contraceptives can be used by women of reproductive age up to the age of 50 years. For those with no contraindications and who would prefer to continue, it can be used up to the age of the menopause because the benefits outweigh the potential risks of use.

6.1.2 Not suitable for the following users

Injectable contraceptives are not suitable (for further information look at UKMEC in *Appendix*) for women with:
- cardiovascular or cerebrovascular disease
- significant multiple risk factors for arterial cardiovascular disease
- current or recent breast cancer
- severe decompensating cirrhosis or liver tumours
- unexplained vaginal bleeding
- at high risk of developing osteoporosis.

6.2 Available injectables in the UK

Details of these are listed in *Table 6.1.*

Table 6.1. Injectables available in the UK

Injectable	Contents	Injection interval and site	Cost per injection
Depo-Provera	Depot medroxyprogesterone acetate (DMPA) 150 mg (as aqueous suspension); should be shaken vigorously prior to use	Given as a deep intramuscular injection every 12 weeks, normally in the upper outer quadrant of the gluteal region. Other sites include lateral thigh and deltoid muscle of upper arm.	£6.01
Sayana Press	DMPA 104 mg (as aqueous suspension); should be shaken vigorously prior to use	Given subcutaneously every 13 weeks in anterior thigh or lower abdomen. It is licensed for pharmacy/self-administration.	£6.90
Noristerat	Norethisterone enanthate (NET-EN) 200 mg (oily injection); should be warmed prior to use	• Given as a deep intramuscular injection every 8 weeks • For short-term, interim contraception but is used infrequently in the UK	£4.05

Data from *BNF*, 2015.

6.3 Mechanism of action

- The main mode of action of DMPA and NET-EN is to inhibit ovulation by suppressing luteinizing hormone (LH) and, to a certain extent, follicle-stimulating hormone (FSH).
- Injectables also alter the cervical mucus, preventing sperm penetration into the upper genital tract.
- Injectables prevent implantation by inducing endometrial atrophy.
- Like other progestogens, injectables modify sperm function and motility.

6.4 Efficacy of injectables

Progestogen-only injectables are highly effective when women receive them on a regular basis, with fewer than 4 women becoming pregnant out of every 1000 over a 2 year period. With imperfect use the typical failure rate in the general population can be as high as 6 in 100 women over 1 year.

6.5 Pros and cons of injectables

6.5.1 Advantages

- Very effective and discreet method of contraception.
- Sayana Press can be self-administered after appropriate training and supervision.

- If pregnancy was to occur during DMPA use there is no evidence of harm to the pregnancy or fetus.
- Non-intercourse related contraceptive method.
- Very safe with no reported attributable deaths.
- Safe for breast-feeding mothers.
- Can be used in women with sickle cell disease with possible reduction in sickle crisis pain.
- Helpful for women with ovulation pain.
- Most women will have infrequent or no periods after 1 year of use and so it is often used for treatment of heavy menstrual bleeding and pain associated with endometriosis.
- Offers most of the non-contraceptive benefits of CHCs, including protection against pelvic inflammatory disease, extra-uterine pregnancies, functional ovarian cysts, fibroid formation.
- May reduce risk of ovarian and endometrial cancer.
- Minimal metabolic effects occur, with recent work reporting no increase in the risk of acute MI, VTE or stroke.

6.5.2 Disadvantages

- A significant number of women fail to return for their second injection, with up to 50% discontinuing its use in the first year. Pre-injection counselling is important to give a realistic picture of potential side-effects, especially menstrual bleeding pattern changes in the first few injection cycles.
- The first few injections of DMPA cause irregular, prolonged vaginal bleeding with increasing episodes of infrequent or no bleeding over time. About one-third of women experience prolonged bleeding (more than 10 days) after receiving their first injection, but 55% are amenorrhoeic at 1 year and 68% at 2 years.
- A possible increase in HIV acquisition/transmission in DMPA users cannot be ruled out and so correct and consistent use of condoms is advised.
- Weight gain is commonly reported in about one-third of women. Obese adolescents (BMI >30 kg/m^2) are more likely to gain weight. In practice this is seen within the first 6 months of administration and weight gain continues over time. On average women may gain up to 3 kg over the first 2 years.
- Some women may complain of mood changes, headaches, loss of libido, bloating and breast tenderness although no causal association has been found.
- It can cause a short delay in the return to a woman's normal fertility.
- There is a possible small increase in the risk of breast cancer diagnosed within the first few years of DMPA use, but this appears to return to background levels following 5 years or more of use. This finding is likely to be due to a screening bias.
- There is a possible increase in the risk of cervical cancer in long-term DMPA users, but this could be due to confounding lifestyle issues.
- Injectables are given intramuscularly and cannot be removed if side-effects occur.

- Injection site reactions are more common with subcutaneous DMPA compared to intramuscular DMPA. Up to 9% of women using subcutaneous DMPA reported indurations, scarring and fat atrophy at the injection site. A small number of women complain of local redness, pain and bruising with either product. Haematoma and abscess formation is a rare event.
- DMPA use results in a small reduction of bone mineral density (BMD), similar to fully breast-feeding for 6 months, which recovers gradually on discontinuation. There are no good data suggesting that DMPA causes osteoporosis or bone fracture. Recent data have suggested that DMPA users are at increased risk of fracture **before** they receive their first injection, implying inherent confounders in those using this method. On discontinuation in adults, BMD recovers to a similar level to never users within 3–5 years. In women under 18 years, BMD recovers more rapidly with it being similar to never users approximately 18 months after stopping. There is no evidence that routinely giving 'add-back' oestrogen to DMPA users or undertaking additional investigations are warranted.

Advice from the MHRA (Department of Health Medicines and Healthcare Products Regulatory Agency) in 2004 stated:
- In adolescents, DMPA may be used as first-line contraception after other methods have been discussed with the patient and considered to be unsuitable or unacceptable.
- In women of all ages, careful re-evaluation of the risks and benefits of treatment should be carried out every 2 years in those who wish to continue its use.
- In women with significant lifestyle and/or medical risk factors for osteoporosis, other methods of contraception should be considered.

6.6 Using injectables

DMPA is given every 13 weeks and a review undertaken at least every 2 years to assess if there have been any changes in the medical history. DMPA can be used until the age of 50 years when a woman may choose an alternative method if there are concerns about her bone health (see *Section 3.2*). On discontinuation it may take up to 12 months before regular menstrual cycles reappear.

There is no evidence that liver enzyme inducing drugs affect the efficacy of DMPA and the injection interval does not need to be shortened. There is a potential loss of efficacy in DMPA users taking ulipristal acetate for emergency contraception or for the management of uterine fibroids. Additional precautions are advised during the time ulipristal acetate is taken and for a further 14 days after it is stopped.

Increasing weight or BMI has not been shown to affect DMPA efficacy. In obese women, deltoid or subcutaneous DMPA administration may be preferred.

6.6.1 Starting regimen

The starting regimen is set out in *Table 6.2*.

Table 6.2. Starting regimen for injectables

Circumstances	Start when?	Extra precautions for 7 days?
Quick start	If no other methods suitable it can be started at any time if it is reasonably certain that the woman is not pregnant (see *Chapter 2*)	Yes
Menstruating	Up to and including day 5	No
	After day 5 of the cycle	Yes
Amenorrhoeic	At any time if it is reasonably certain that the woman is not pregnant	Yes
Following first or second trimester abortion or miscarriage	Within 5 days	No
	After 5 days	Yes
Following emergency contraception	After taking levonorgestrel 1500 mcg	Yes
	After taking ulipristal acetate 30 mg	Yes – start 5 whole days after taking ulipristal acetate 30 mg; abstinence or use of condoms needed for a further 7 days
Post-partum, whether breast-feeding or bottle feeding	Before and including day 21	No; ideally delay to day 21 because possible risk of prolonged bleeding
	After day 21 in women who are menstruating	Yes, as for women having menstrual cycles
	After day 21 in those not menstruating	Yes, as for those women who are amenorrhoeic
Switching from other hormonal methods (other than IUS or POP)	Immediate start	No
Switching from an IUS or POP	Immediate start	Yes for 7 days until ovulation suppression can be assured or continue using an IUS/taking POP for a further 7 days
Switching from a non-hormonal method (other than IUD)	Up to and including day 5	No
	After day 5	Yes
Switching from an IUD	Give the injection up to and including day 5 of cycle; IUD can be removed at the same time	No
	Any other time and unprotected sex has occurred in the last 7 days	Yes; IUD should be continued for the next 7 days

6.6.2 Advice about late injections

Recent guidance states that both Depo-Provera and Sayana Press can now be administered every 13 weeks. No action is required for either preparation until 14 weeks or more has lapsed since the last injection.

- If a woman presents within 14 weeks of receiving her last injection then the next injection is administered and no further action needs to be taken.
- If more than 14 weeks has elapsed since the last injection, but no unprotected sex has occurred from 14 weeks onwards, then the next injection is given and additional contraception or abstinence advised for the next 7 days.
- If more than 14 weeks has elapsed since the last injection, and unprotected sex **has only** occurred in the last 5 days, exclude the risk of pregnancy, consider emergency contraception, give the next injection and advise additional contraception or abstinence for the next 7 days. A pregnancy test should be repeated in 3 weeks.
- If more than 14 weeks has elapsed since the last injection, and unprotected sex has occurred from 14 weeks onwards for more than 5 days, then pregnancy should be excluded, the next injection is given and additional contraception or abstinence for the next 7 days. A further pregnancy test is advised in 3 weeks.

6.7 Routine follow-up

Women are advised to return when their next injection is due, unless troublesome side-effects occur, when an earlier appointment is indicated. At that visit enquiries should be made concerning sexual and medical health, changes in bleeding pattern and presence of nuisance side-effects. The MHRA guidance should be followed.

DMPA users are responsible for making repeat appointments but some practices send reminder text messages and others suggest mobile phone apps.

6.8 Return to fertility

There may be a delay to the return of fertility, with mean time to ovulation being 5.3 months after the preceding injection. Fertility rates by 2 years are similar to non-hormonal contraceptive methods.

6.9 Managing side-effects

6.9.1 Prolonged and frequent bleeding

- Women should be counselled about the changes in menstrual pattern before DMPA is administered. Prolonged bleeding/spotting is commonly reported during the first injection cycle.
- If prolonged and/or frequent bleeding is reported to be a problem:
  - exclude gynaecological pathology by taking a clinical and lifestyle history enquiring about abdominal/pelvic pain, dyspareunia, vaginal discharge, dysuria, post-coital bleeding, new sexual partners

- o a pelvic examination is required if irregular bleeding has occurred for more than 3 months, other symptoms are present, a previous medical treatment has failed or the woman is anxious
  - o exclude pregnancy in sexually active women
  - o perform STI screening in those at risk
  - o for those eligible to participate in the NHS Cervical Screening programme review cervical screening history and perform a cervical screen only if it is due.
- Treatment may stop a bleeding episode but confers no long-term benefit, including:
  - o prescribing a COC (30 mcg ethinylestradiol with levonorgestrel) for up to 3 months cyclically or continuously (unlicensed), if there are no contraindications. Depending on clinical judgement, it may be used longer term; however, there are no long-term safety data available
  - o prescribing tranexamic acid 250 mg four times a day for 5 days or mefenamic acid 500 mg up to three times a day for 5 days to reduce bleeding in the short term
  - o reducing the injection interval by 2 weeks if bleeding occurs towards the end of the injection cycle.

6.9.2 Weight gain

- Advise women that two out of three women do not gain weight with DMPA.
- Weight gain with DMPA is more likely to occur in women with a previous history of labile weight changes.
- Keep to a healthy Mediterranean diet containing only complex carbohydrates.
- Women who gain more than 5% of their baseline body weight in the first 6 months are likely to continue to gain weight.

6.10 Myths and misconceptions

- **DMPA reduces your fertility** – DMPA may delay the return of a woman's fertility but does not affect pregnancy rates 2 years after discontinuation.
- **DMPA increases the risk of a premature menopause** – DMPA administration may stop periods but these return within the first year of discontinuation. It does not bring the age of the menopause forward for women.
- **DMPA makes you fat** – there is evidence that some DMPA users gain weight but most either stay the same or lose weight. Those who gain weight often say that they feel hungrier and are therefore eating more. If a woman has a tendency to gain weight then she should be advised to watch her diet when using DMPA. If she gains a significant amount of weight in the first 6 months then she may wish to choose a different method of contraception.
- **DMPA is unsafe as it causes osteoporosis** – there is no evidence that DMPA alone causes osteoporosis or osteoporotic fractures. For the majority of women the change in BMD is of little clinical significance. It is important to take a careful history to exclude any potential risks to bone health before it is prescribed and at 2 yearly intervals.

EXAMPLE

A 24 year old woman has been using DMPA for 3 years. She wants a baby and stopped having DMPA injections 18 months ago but has still not had a period.

What should you do?

1. As it has been 12 months since her last injection, check other causes for secondary amenorrhoea including undertaking blood tests to check FSH, LH, oestradiol, thyroid function tests, prolactin.
2. Check her BMI.
3. Perform a pregnancy test.
4. If all investigations are normal refer her to a gynaecologist who specializes in fertility issues because she may need ovulation induction.

References

British National Formulary, September 2014–March 2015.

eMC: SPC Depo-Provera 150 mg/ml injection
[www.medicines.org.uk/emc/medicine/11121 – accessed April 2016]

eMC: SPC Sayana Press 104 mg/0.65 ml suspension for injection
[www.medicines.org.uk/emc/medicine/27798/SPC/SAYANA+PRESS+104+mg+0.65+ml+suspension+for+injection/ – accessed April 2016]

FSRH (2015) *Problematic Bleeding with Hormonal Contraception*. Clinical Effectiveness Unit.
[www.fsrh.org/documents/ceuguidanceproblematicbleedinghormonalcontraception/ – accessed June 2016]

FSRH (2015) Progestogen-only Injectable Contraception. Clinical Effectiveness Unit.
[www.fsrh.org/documents/cec-ceu-guidance-injectables-dec-2014/ – accessed June 2016]

Lanza L.L., *et al.* (2013) Use of depot medroxyprogesterone acetate contraception and incidence of bone fracture. *Obstet Gynecol.* **121:** 593–600.

Office for National Statistics (2009) Opinions Survey Report No. 41 *Contraception and Sexual Health*, 2008/09.

UKMEC (2016) *UK Medical Eligibility Criteria for Contraceptive Use*
[www.fsrh.org/standards-and-guidance/uk-medical-eligibility-criteria-for-contraceptive-use/ – accessed June 2016]

Chapter 7
Contraceptive implant

A contraceptive implant offers an alternative way of delivering hormones providing long-acting, low-dose, reversible contraception. It is one of the most effective contraceptives licensed to provide contraception for 3 years with 2% of women in the UK using this method.

In 1999 a single progestogen-only implant, Implanon, was launched containing 68 mg etonogestrel, the active metabolite of desogestrel. Nexplanon, a bioequivalent implant with additional barium sulphate to make it radiopaque, is now available. It also has a new applicator to facilitate single-handed, subdermal insertion.

Norplant, the levonorgestrel implant, consists of six rods inserted subdermally on the inner aspect of the upper arm. It was available in the UK from 1993 until 1999, but UK healthcare professionals may still see women from sub-Saharan Africa using this multi-rod contraceptive system, or the two-rod levonorgestrel system, Jadelle.

7.1 Potential users

7.1.1 Most appropriate users

There are few contraindications to its use and no age limit so it is suitable for the majority of women.

7.1.2 Not suitable for the following users

The implant may not be effective in women taking liver enzyme inducing drugs and should be avoided in women who:
- have had a hormone-dependent tumour (e.g. breast cancer) in the last 5 years
- have severe decompensating liver disease or liver tumours
- are sensitive to any of the components of the etonogestrel implant
- are currently using an etonogestrel implant and develop ischaemic heart or cerebrovascular disease
- have unexplained vaginal bleeding.

7.2 Available implants in the UK

Nexplanon, which contains 68 mg etonogestrel, is licensed to provide effective contraception for 3 years. It is inserted subdermally on the inner side of the upper arm. It costs £79.46 and is the only implant available in the UK.

7.3 Mechanism of action

- The etonogestrel implant inhibits ovulation by suppressing luteinizing hormone. However, up to 5% of users may ovulate in the third year.
- Implants also alter the cervical mucus, inhibiting sperm penetration and thereby preventing fertilization.
- Implants prevent implantation by inducing endometrial atrophy.
- Implants may modify sperm function and motility.

7.4 Efficacy of implants

This is a highly effective method of contraception with less than 1 woman in every 1000 users becoming pregnant over a 3 year period.

Liver enzyme inducing drugs will reduce the efficacy of progestogen implants and so additional contraception is required when there is concomitant use with certain anti-epileptic medication, ART and enzyme-inducing antibiotics such as rifampicin (see *Chapter 3* for drug interactions).

There have been concerns that progestogen implants are less effective in heavier women because etonogestrel levels fall with increasing weight, although they stay within the therapeutic range. There is evidence that these implants are effective in women weighing up to 149 kg. Although the manufacturer suggests replacing the implant earlier in the third year for such women there is little evidence to support this, although it should be considered if the woman starts to return to a regular cycle in that period.

7.5 Pros and cons of contraceptive implants

7.5.1 Advantages

- Long-lasting, effective, immediately reversible contraceptive method.
- It can be used by women who have previously experienced an ectopic pregnancy because it is highly effective and its main mechanism of action is to suppress ovulation. The risk of ectopic pregnancy is very small.
- No effect on future fertility.
- In the rare event of an unplanned pregnancy, there is no adverse effect on the pregnancy or fetus.
- Non-intercourse related method.
- Free from oestrogen side-effects.
- High user acceptability following pre-insertion counselling, with first year continuation rates of over 70%.

- Requires little medical attention other than at insertion and removal.
- May reduce ovulation pain.
- Reduced incidence of dysmenorrhoea in women with or without endometriosis.
- Reduced total menstrual blood loss in implant users.
- No evidence to suggest adverse effect on bone mineral density.
- Can be used by those where synthetic oestrogen is contraindicated, including women complaining of migraine with aura.
- Does not adversely affect cardiovascular risk factors with no increased risk of VTE, MI or stroke in implant users.
- Has minimal effects on glucose metabolism and liver function.

7.5.2 Disadvantages

- Unpredictable and irregular bleeding patterns are common in implant users, with the bleeding pattern experienced during the first 3 months being broadly predictive of future bleeding patterns.
- In the first two years of implant use, approximately 22% have amenorrhoea, 33% infrequent bleeding, 7% frequent bleeding and/or prolonged bleeding (18%) per 90-day reference period.
- Enlarged ovarian follicles >2.5 cm may be found in 5–25% of Nexplanon users. These are rarely symptomatic and tend to disappear over time. Women with persistent follicles are more likely to complain of prolonged bleeding.
- Incidence of progestogen side-effects with Nexplanon are similar to other progestogen-only methods and include headache, weight gain, acne, loss of libido, mood changes. No causal association has been found.
- Acne may improve, stay the same or worsen with the use of the implant.
- Fat atrophy may occur over the site of the implant.
- Insertion of implants requires a minor operative procedure under local anaesthetic by trained healthcare professionals.
- Non-palpable implants have been reported in about 1 in 1000 insertions and are related to poor insertion technique. Very occasionally, deep insertion of the implant has resulted in damage to the neurovascular bundle. Referral to an 'expert' centre is advised for implant location using ultrasound scanning before removal.
- In cases where the implant cannot be located by ultrasound scanning or X-ray, etonogestrel assays may be required.
- Some women report mild discomfort and bruising following insertion or removal of the implants.
- Infection at the insertion or removal site, irritation over the implant, breakage of the implant, local fibrosis around the implant, migration of the implants and scarring do occur, but only rarely.
- For some women contraceptive implants may not be a suitable method because discontinuation is not under their control.
- There have been no studies looking at progestogen-only implant use and risk of breast cancer and so there is insufficient evidence to indicate any increased risk.
- There have been no studies investigating progestogen-only implant use and gynaecological cancers and so there is insufficient evidence to indicate any increased risk.

7.6 Practical aspects

7.6.1 Implant starting regimen

Table 7.1 provides details as to when implants can be inserted under a range of circumstances.

Table 7.1. Implant starting regimes

Circumstances	Start when?	Extra precautions for 7 days?
Quick starting	At any time if it is reasonably certain that the woman is not pregnant	Yes
Menstruating	Up to and including day 5	No
	After day 5 if it is reasonably certain that the woman is not pregnant or at risk of pregnancy	Yes
Amenorrhoeic	Any time if it is reasonably certain that the woman is not pregnant or at risk of pregnancy	Yes
After a first or second trimester abortion or miscarriage	Within 5 days	No
	After 5 days if it is reasonably certain that she is not pregnant or at risk of pregnancy	Yes
Post-partum	Before or on day 21 post-partum	No
Breast-feeding or bottle feeding	From day 22 onwards	Yes (unless menstruation has recommenced, when it can be fitted up to day 5 of the cycle)
Following oral emergency contraception	Immediately following levonorgestrel 1500 mcg	Yes
	Immediately following ulipristal acetate	Yes – start 5 whole days after taking ulipristal acetate 30 mg; abstinence or use of condoms needed for a further 7 days
Switching from CHC	Immediate start	No
	Week 1 following the hormone-free interval	Yes – if unprotected sex has occurred in the hormone-free interval the CHC should be restarted for at least 7 days
	Week 2–3 of combined pill, patch, vaginal ring	No, as long as CHC has been used consistently and correctly
Switching from an injectable	Immediately within 14 weeks of last injection	No
	14 weeks +1 day or more	Yes and consider EC if unprotected sex has occurred after 14 weeks

Circumstances	Start when?	Extra precautions for 7 days?
Switching from a POP or LNG-IUS	Any time	7 days of additional contraception or continue to use POP or LNG-IUS for a further 7 days until ovulation is suppressed
Switching from a non-hormonal method including a copper IUD	Up to and including day 5 of cycle	No
	After day 5 or amenorrhoeic	Yes; if unprotected sex has occurred within the previous 7 days IUD should be retained for a further 7 days

7.6.2 Insertion of the implant

Those offering implant insertion and removal should be appropriately trained clinicians holding an up-to-date FSRH Letter of Competence in Subdermal Contraceptive Implant Techniques or have equivalent competencies. They should maintain their competence and regularly update their theoretical and practical knowledge.

The location of the insertion is shown in *Figure 7.1* and the basic technique in *Figure 7.2*.
- Etonogestrel implants are either fitted using an aseptic or 'no touch' technique, with the woman either lying down or sitting with her arm resting on a support.
- The non-dominant arm is externally rotated.
- Local anaesthetic with or without adrenaline is injected subdermally. Check that the implant is in the insertion needle, then insert the implant just under the skin one-third of the way up the inner aspect of the upper arm, away from the sulcus of the biceps and triceps (*Figure 7.2*). Addition of a vasoconstrictor reduces blood loss and may be useful in women taking anticoagulants or where a deep implant is planned.
- Once the implant has been fitted its position should be confirmed by both the clinician and patient. The applicator is designed to reduce the chance of non-insertion. At this stage the needle should be fully retracted inside the applicator's handle.

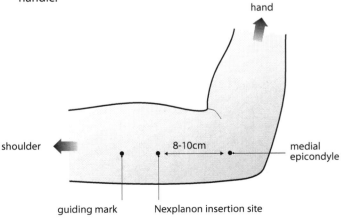

Figure 7.1. Nexplanon insertion site.

- ○ If the implant cannot be felt easily, the woman should be advised to use additional contraception and return in a week when there is less swelling and bruising. If it is still not palpable then the guidance for managing deep implants below should be followed.
- The arm is then dressed and advice regarding wound care given.

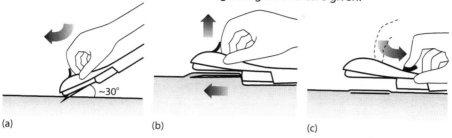

(a)   (b)   (c)

Figure 7.2. Nexplanon insertion. (a) Piercing of the skin; (b) subdermal insertion of the applicator needle; (c) retraction of the slider to withdraw the needle, placing the implant subdermally.

7.6.3 Removal of implant

A woman can decide to have the implant removed at any point following its insertion – she should not be coerced to keep it. Discuss the reasons for its removal and whether there may be options for treating any side-effects such as erratic bleeding pattern, headaches, etc. Future contraceptive/preconception plans should be covered during the consultation. To avoid an unplanned pregnancy another contraceptive method should be started immediately following removal of the implant (see 'switching advice for individual methods' in *Chapters 4–9*).

The removal procedure is outlined below and illustrated in *Figure 7.3*.
- The skin over the distal end of the implant is marked with water-soluble marker pen and local anaesthetic injected just under its tip.
- A small longitudinal incision is made in the skin and the implant is pushed through the incision using the 'pop out' method.

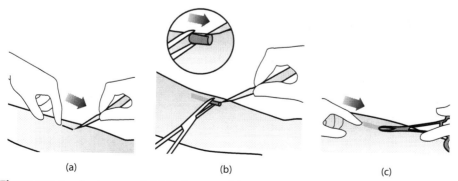

(a)   (b)   (c)

Figure 7.3. Implant removal. (a) Make a small longitudinal incision over the distal end of the implant; (b) clean away the connective tissue; (c) remove the implant.

- Connective tissue is cleaned away from the tip of the implant and then it is removed.
- The small wound can be closed with paper sutures and then dressed.
- If a further implant is requested, this can be inserted through the same incision, ensuring that its position is subdermal.
- Insertion and removal counselling/procedures should be clearly documented in the clinical record.

7.6.4 Management of deep or bent implants

- Impalpable implants normally result from poor insertion technique and frequently occur at the time of removing and reinserting new implants. Rarely, nerve or vascular damage can occur with deep implant insertions or problematic removals, with intravascular migration to the pulmonary tree occasionally reported. Beware of women with thin arms because the needle tip can be accidentally placed under the muscle fascia, resulting in an intramuscular insertion.
- Implant migration up or down the arm is more commonly seen where the implant is deeply placed in muscle and in women who try to move the implant under their skin.
- If an implant cannot easily be felt then the woman should be advised to abstain from sex or use an additional method of contraception. In these situations:
  - Do not attempt removal.
  - If the implant is Nexplanon, arrange an X-ray of the arm. If the implant can be seen then it will still be effective as a contraceptive and it does not need to be removed unless there is discomfort/pain.
  - If removal is requested by the woman or it needs to be changed, refer to the regional centre providing deep implant removals. Further information is available from manufacturers (www.msd-uk.com).
  - High resolution ultrasound will be used to locate the implant and it is normally removed through a small incision. If the implant cannot be located the manufacturer can arrange an etonogestrel assay in the Netherlands. If this demonstrates etonogestrel in the body then a chest X-ray should be arranged.
- Implants are flexible and can be bent or fractured by women, without apparently affecting their efficacy; they can remain *in situ*.

7.6.5 Advice about late removal of implants

Nexplanon is licensed to provide contraception for 3 years. If it is changed within the 3 year period no abstinence from sex or additional contraceptive method is required.

If more than 3 years has elapsed the chance of pregnancy is very small. However, a urinary pregnancy test should be performed and women advised to abstain or use condoms consistently and correctly for a further week. The pregnancy test is then repeated after 3 weeks and the implant changed. Additional precautions are required for a further 3 weeks.

7.7 Routine follow-up

If the implant has been fitted following the 'quick-start' guidance (see *Table 7.1*) a pregnancy test should be performed 3 weeks later. Otherwise there is no need to see the woman again unless:

- she has concerns
- the implant needs to be changed
- the implant cannot be felt
- there is pain or irritation over the implant
- there are signs of infection, the implant appears broken or the woman is worried about pregnancy.

7.8 Return to fertility

Following implant removal there is an immediate return to a woman's pre-existing fertility (depending upon her age), with etonogestrel levels undetectable at 1 week. Most women start to ovulate within 3 weeks of implant removal.

7.9 Managing troublesome side-effects

7.9.1 Bleeding problems

- Take a careful medical and relationship history.
- Exclude STIs and any gynaecology pathology.
- Check, where applicable, that cervical screening is up-to-date.
- Perform a pelvic examination if there are other symptoms including dysmenorrhoea, dyspareunia, vaginal discharge, dysuria.
- Perform a pelvic examination if unexplained troublesome bleeding has persisted for more than 6 months or a medical treatment has failed to stop a bleeding episode. Treatment options to stop a bleeding episode include:
  - using a continuous or cyclically combined hormonal contraceptive (pill, patch or ring) for 3 months (outside of the product licence)
  - tranexamic acid 250 mg four a day for 5 days
  - mefenamic acid 500 mg up to 3 times a day for 5 days
  - anecdotally, one desogestrel POP daily or therapeutic doses of progestogen for up to 3 months (medroxyprogesterone acetate 10 mg up to 3 times a day continuously or for 21 days with a 7 day break).
- There is no evidence that these treatments confer a long-term benefit.

7.9.2 Headaches

Headaches are commonly reported by the general population with no causal link found with implant use. Suggest paracetamol/ibuprofen as appropriate.

7.9.3 Acne

Women switching from combined hormonal contraceptives to progestogen-only methods, such as implants, may complain of acne as sex hormone binding globulin levels fall and resultant free testosterone levels rise. Studies have shown that acne may improve, worsen or remain the same in implant users. Standard topical acne therapies can be tried.

7.10 Myths and misconceptions

- **Implants make you fat** – there is no evidence that implant users gain any more weight than their peers.
- **Implants are difficult to remove** – if they are fitted correctly in the subdermal plane, removal should be straightforward.
- **Implants make you bleed all the time** – most women are satisfied with the bleeding pattern, but the key is to give a realistic picture before fitting the implant. Unfortunately, some may assume they will have very little bleeding if their friends with implants have infrequent periods.

EXAMPLE

A 20 year old secretary has just had her implant changed and feels that she has more bloating with the new implant. She has also found that her menstrual bleeding pattern has changed as she is having more infrequent bleeds.

What do you advise?

1. Take a medical and relationship history.
2. Check that she had her implant changed before 3 years.
3. Perform a pregnancy test and STI screen.
4. If all is fine, remind the patient that a new implant releases 50% more hormone when compared to her previous implant that had been in place for 3 years, which explains why she has noticed a change in her bleeding pattern. The bloating should improve over the first few months but she is likely to continue with infrequent periods.

References

British National Formulary, September 2014–March 2015.

eMC: SPC Nexplanon 68 mg implant for subdermal use [www.medicines.org.uk/emc/medicine/23824/SPC/Nexplanon+68+mg+implant+ for+subdermal+use/ – accessed April 2016]

FSRH (2014) *Progestogen-only Implants*. Clinical Effectiveness Unit. [www.fsrh.org/documents/cec-ceu-guidance-implants-feb-2014/ – accessed June 2016]

FSRH (2015) *Problematic Bleeding with Hormonal Contraception*. Clinical Effectiveness Unit. [www.fsrh.org/documents/ceuguidanceproblematicbleedinghormonalcontraception/ – accessed June 2016]

Office for National Statistics (2009) Opinions Survey Report No. 41 *Contraception and Sexual Health*, 2008/09.

UKMEC (2016) *UK Medical Eligibility Criteria for Contraceptive Use* [www.fsrh.org/standards-and-guidance/uk-medical-eligibility-criteria-for-contraceptive-use/ – accessed June 2016]

Chapter 8
Intrauterine system

Intrauterine contraception (IUC) includes intrauterine systems (IUS) and intrauterine devices (IUD). IUCs provide cost-effective, reliable, long-acting and reversible contraception. While an IUS may be more suitable for women who have heavy bleeding, an IUD provides effective contraception for those seeking an effective non-hormonal method. However, in many cases either an IUS or an IUD will be a suitable option for women to consider.

For simplicity and ease of access to information the IUS will be discussed in this chapter and the IUD in *Chapter 9*, although many of the issues discussed are applicable to all IUC methods.

There are three levonorgestrel-containing intrauterine systems (IUS) available in the UK. The first two contain 52 mg of levonorgestrel (IUS-52 – Mirena and Levosert). Mirena has been available in the UK since May 1995 and Levosert since April 2015. The third, containing 13.5 mg of levonorgestrel (IUS-13.5 – Jaydess), was launched in April 2014. Both IUS-52 IUSs are also licensed for the treatment of heavy menstrual bleeding; however, only Mirena is licensed as the progestogen component of hormone replacement therapy.

8.1 Potential users

8.1.1 Most appropriate users

- For the majority of women the benefits of the IUS outweigh the risks.
- The IUS is suitable for all women of reproductive age until contraception is no longer required, providing there are no contraindications (see UKMEC in *Appendix*).
- An IUS can be used in women who have not had a previous pregnancy and continuation rates are similar for parous and nulliparous women.
- As the IUS provides immediately reversible contraception it is well suited to women wishing to space pregnancies.

- An IUS offers long-term effective contraception and is a suitable alternative to sterilization for women who have completed their families.
- An IUS is the first-line medical treatment for heavy menstrual bleeding and will reduce dysmenorrhoea.
- An IUS can be used for women with undetectable β-hCG and a history of trophoblastic disease.

8.1.2 Not suitable for the following users

The IUS is not suitable (for further information see UKMEC in *Appendix*) for women with:
- unexplained vaginal bleeding
- post-partum women between 48 hours and 4 weeks post-delivery
- post-partum or post-abortion sepsis
- persistently elevated β-hCG or malignant disease
- cervical cancer awaiting treatment
- endometrial cancer
- current pelvic inflammatory disease
- current chlamydia or gonorrhoea (unless the infection is asymptomatic and treatment is given. Decision whether or not to fit should be made on a case-by-case basis)
- known pelvic tuberculosis
- known serious cardiac conditions or arrhythmias where a vasovagal collapse may have serious consequences
- HIV positive with a CD4 count <200 cells/mm³.

8.2 Available intrauterine systems in the UK

These are detailed in *Table 8.1*.

Table 8.1. IUS available in the UK

Trade name	Hormonal content	Size of device	Duration of use	Cost
Mirena	52 mg (20 mcg released daily, reducing to 10 mcg per day at 5 years)	32 × 32 mm Diameter of insertion tube – 4.4 mm	5 years	£88.00
Levosert	52 mg (20 mcg released daily, reducing to 12 mcg per day at 3 years)	32 x 32 mm Diameter of insertion tube – 4.8 mm	3 years (trials on-going)	£66.00
Jaydess	13.5 mg (14 mcg released daily for first 24 days, reducing to 5 mcg per day at 3 years)	28 × 30 mm Diameter of insertion tube – 3.8 mm	3 years	£69.22

Data from *British National Formulary*, 2015; SPC Levosert, 2015.

8.3 Mechanism of action

- The IUS exerts its main contraceptive action pre-fertilization by altering the cervical mucus and utero-tubal fluid, which inhibits sperm penetration and migration.

- The IUS down-regulates oestrogen and progesterone receptors within the endometrium, making it relatively insensitive to circulating oestrogen. This prevents endometrial proliferation causing atrophic changes to occur within a month of insertion. This will prevent implantation if fertilization occurs.
- The progestogen may affect sperm motility and function, preventing fertilization.
- Ovulation may be suppressed in a small number of users in the first year, possibly by reducing the pre-ovulatory LH surge. However, serum oestradiol levels are not reduced.

8.4 Efficacy

- The IUS-52 (Mirena) has a failure rate of up to 2 in 1000 over 5 years, with cumulative pregnancy rates of less than 1% at 5 years. Levosert appears to have a similar failure rate although data are limited.
- The IUS-13.5 (Jaydess) has a similar failure rate of 0.33 pregnancies per 100 women-years, with a cumulative failure rate of 0.9% over 3 years.

8.5 Pros and cons of IUS

8.5.1 Advantages

- Long-acting and independent of sexual intercourse.
- No known drug interactions.
- Highly effective contraceptive (as effective as female sterilization) with an immediate return to fertility after removal. Increasing use of LARCs such as the IUS has led to a fall in requests for female sterilization in the UK.
- Reduces menstrual blood loss in women with no period problems. About one-quarter of women will be amenorrhoeic by year 3 when using the IUS-52 (Mirena).
- IUS-52 reduces heavy menstrual bleeding by about 97% after 12 months, with an associated improvement in haemoglobin and serum ferritin; this has led to gynaecologists performing fewer hysterectomies in the UK. It can be used in women with coagulation disorders or taking anticoagulants. The IUS-13.5 also reduces menstrual bleeding but to a lesser extent.
- Long-term use may prevent fibroid formation.
- Reduces heavy menstrual bleeding associated with the presence of fibroids and adenomyosis.
- Reduces the incidence of dysmenorrhoea in the general population and for women with adenomyosis.
- May be a useful medical treatment for women suffering from endometriosis, with significant improvements in severity and frequency of pain/menstrual symptoms. It is also a good maintenance therapy following conservative surgery for endometriosis.
- No evidence that the IUS affects serum oestradiol levels and BMD.
- Reduces the risk of ectopic pregnancy and can be used in women with a past history of extra-uterine pregnancies.
- Reduces the incidence of pelvic inflammatory disease.

- Mirena (IUS-52) is licensed to be used as the progestogenic component of hormone replacement therapy.
- May protect against the development of endometrial hyperplasia. The IUS-52 (Mirena) has been shown to resolve endometrial hyperplasia without atypia in 92% of cases and endometrial hyperplasia with atypia in 67% of women. It should not be used in women with early endometrial cancer.
- Has a high user acceptance rate with 3 year continuation rates over 70%.

8.5.2 Disadvantages

- Can cause irregular/prolonged bleeding in the first 3 months in women using the IUS for contraception. Prolonged bleeding/spotting (6 months or more following fitting) may occur in those with heavy menstrual bleeding with or without fibroids. Pre-insertion counselling is important and a realistic picture, describing this menstrual disturbance, must be given.
- The IUS may be expelled or displaced in about 4–6% of cases, particularly if intra-cavity fibroids are present or in women complaining of heavy menstrual loss.
- The fitting may be painful.
- Failure to fit the IUS can occur in 1–2% of cases as a result of pain during insertion or difficulties passing the sound or device through the cervix. This may be due to an anatomical anomaly or operator technique. The woman should be offered an alternative appointment with another more experienced fitter. An alternative contraceptive method should be provided in the interim.
- Like other IUCs there is a small increased risk of pelvic infection immediately after fitting (within the first 20 days), particularly in young women. Therefore those at risk of STIs should be screened prior to fitting (see *Chapter 9*).
- A small number of women may develop functional ovarian cysts but these tend to resolve over 6 months or so and rarely require surgical intervention. Often they are asymptomatic and are more common in users of IUS-52 rather than IUS-13.5.
- Rare complications such as perforation of the uterus/cervix may occur (less than 2 per 1000 devices fitted) but this is more common in breast-feeding women.
- Some progestogenic symptoms may occur in the first few months following fitting, such as breast tenderness, bloating or acne. These symptoms tend to improve with time.
- In the event of IUS failure, between 25% and 50% of these pregnancies will be ectopic, although the overall risk of ectopic pregnancy is lower than in the general population. For the IUS-52 the ectopic rate is 0.02 per 100 women-years and for the IUS-13.5 the ectopic rate is 0.11 per 100 women-years.
- The IUS cannot be used as an emergency form of contraception.

8.6 Counselling

- A medical history should be taken to ensure medical eligibility, along with comprehensive counselling encompassing the advantages, disadvantages, side-effects (including perforation and expulsion rates), and details of the fitting procedure.

- Effective counselling helps women to choose the most appropriate contraceptive method.
- Women should be advised to abstain from sex following a normal period or use a bridging method until the IUS can be fitted.
- Take an STI history and undertake screening (chlamydia screening as a minimum) in women under 25 years old, or in women older than 25 with a new partner or more than 1 partner in the preceding 12 months. The IUS can be fitted on the same day as counselling and STI screening in asymptomatic women who are not at risk of pregnancy.
- There is no need to screen for bacterial vaginosis or candida infections.
- If the IUS is being used for heavy menstrual bleeding or dysmenorrhoea, further investigation such as full blood count, ultrasound scan and endometrial biopsy may be indicated.
- Women should be advised to seek help if they have heavy bleeding or severe pain after the IUS is fitted, if they develop an abnormal smelly vaginal discharge or if they think they are pregnant. If a pregnancy is confirmed by a urinary/serum pregnancy test then its site should be ascertained by ultrasound scan.
- Provide written information about the method, such as the Family Planning Association leaflet, available at www.fpa.org.uk. *Table 8.2* provides a summary of topics to be included during discussion and in written information.

Table 8.2. Topics to cover during counselling and in written information

Topics
Advantages and disadvantages
Efficacy and mechanism of action
Perforation rate – up to 2 per 1000; this rate is increased 6-fold in breast-feeding women within 36 weeks of delivery (Heinemann *et al.*, 2015a)
Expulsion rate – 1 in 20; highest in the first 3 months post-insertion and during menstruation
Infection – 6-fold increased risk of PID in the first 20 days post-insertion, after which risk is low and remains low
Pregnancy and ectopic risk – pregnancy risk less than 1% a year and overall ectopic pregnancy risk very low, but if pregnancy occurs 25–50% may be ectopic
Bleeding pattern changes – 1 in 4 women using IUS-52 (Mirena) experience amenorrhoea (this increases to 60% with a subsequent IUS); 1 in 10 women using IUS-13.5 experience amenorrhoea
Hormonal side-effects – more common in the first few months of use and decrease over time; these include breast tenderness, headaches, acne and mood changes
Bridging contraception until the IUS is fitted – abstain or use effective method of contraception

8.7 IUS starting regimen

This is described in *Table 8.3*.

Table 8.3. Starting regimens for IUS in a variety of circumstances

Circumstances	Start when?	Extra precautions for 7 days?
Menstruating	Up to and including day 7 (avoiding insertion when menstrual flow is heavy, to reduce chance of subsequent expulsion)	No
	After day 7 of the cycle, as long as it is reasonable certain that the woman is not pregnant	Yes
Amenorrhoeic	Any time if it is reasonably certain that the woman is not pregnant	Yes
Post-abortion or miscarriage (<24 weeks of gestation)	Within 7 days of event	No
	After 7 days of event	Yes
Post-partum Breast-feeding or bottle feeding	Within the first 48 hours post-partum	No
	After day 28 (including following a Caesarean section) providing fitter is reasonably certain woman is not pregnant	Yes
Switching from other hormonal methods (other than IUS)	Immediately after last day of active hormone for CHC users	No
	If inserted after day 1 of hormone-free interval or in week 1 of CHC cycle	Yes; continue the CHC for 7 days or use alternative contraception for 7 days
	Up to 3 years post insertion of progestogen-only implant	No
	After 3 years post insertion of progestogen-only implant	Yes (7 days) as long as it is reasonably certain that the woman is not pregnant
	Less than 14 weeks post progestogen-only injectable	No
	More than 14 weeks post progestogen-only injectable (as long as reasonably certain woman is not pregnant)	Yes; additional method such as barrier for 7 days
	For POP users insertion can occur at any time	Yes; continue POP for 7 days
Switching from a non-hormonal method (other than IUD)	Up to and including day 7	No
	After day 7 if reasonably certain the woman is not pregnant	Yes

Circumstances	Start when?	Extra precautions for 7 days?
Switching from an IUD or changing an IUS	Insert the IUS up to and including day 7 of a cycle	No
	After day 7, advise no sexual intercourse for 7 days prior to the IUS fitting	Yes
	If the woman is using an IUS and is amenorrhoeic or has irregular bleeds, advise no sexual intercourse for 7 days prior to the changing of the IUS	No
	If insertion of Mirena IUS-52 occurred 5–7 years ago in a woman under age 45, removal and re-insertion may occur immediately if pregnancy test is negative	Yes for 7 days
	If insertion of Mirena IUS-52 occurred >7 years ago in woman under age 45, replacement should be delayed for at least 3 weeks after last UPSI and at which time a pregnancy test should be undertaken	Yes for 7 days

8.8 IUS insertion

- Undertake a bimanual examination to assess the size, position, shape and motility of the uterus and exclude pathology.
- Using a non-touch (aseptic) technique insert a speculum, hold cervix with forceps (Allis or tenaculum) and apply gentle traction to straighten out uterine flexion and reduce the risk of perforation.
- Assess cavity length with a uterine sound.
- Insert the IUS following the product recommendations, ensuring final placement is at the fundus of the uterus. Each product has a slightly different insertion technique, therefore it is important for fitters to be appropriately trained.
- Trim the threads so that they are 3 cm long outside the external os of the cervix.

8.9 Post IUS insertion advice

- Instructions are given on how and when to check IUS threads. Women should seek advice if the threads feel longer than normal, if they are unable to feel the threads, or if the tip of the device is felt.
- Post-insertion pain is common in the first few days up to a week post-insertion. If this does not resolve with simple analgesics women are advised to return for assessment.
- If there are symptoms suggestive of infection, such as foul-smelling discharge, abdominal pain and fever, advice and assessment should be undertaken by a general practitioner or at a local sexual health clinic.

8.10 Routine follow-up

- A 6 week follow-up appointment for assessment of bleeding, infection, expulsion and perforation is routinely undertaken. During this consultation women are asked about bleeding and if any pain has been experienced. In addition, women

are asked if they have felt the IUS threads and if the threads can be felt during sex; if this is the case then the threads should be shortened. The woman is examined to check the thread length, ensure that the IUS stem cannot be felt in the cervical canal and that cervical excitation is not present.
- Routine yearly medical checks are not required. Women should be advised to return if they are unable to feel the IUS threads, have unexplained abdominal pain or have experienced unscheduled bleeding after the first 3–6 months.
- Additional follow-up can be undertaken if the woman has any further concerns.

8.11 Return to fertility and device removal
- Following removal of the IUS there is no delay in return to fertility.
- To avoid an unplanned pregnancy the IUS should be removed when there has been no unprotected sex for the preceding 7 days.

8.12 Managing side-effects and complications

8.12.1 Spotting or bleeding
- Irregular, light or prolonged bleeding commonly occurs in IUS users, particularly in the first 3–6 months of use, and typically settles without treatment.
- Histologically large thin-walled blood vessels appear within an atrophic endometrium which may explain the unscheduled bleeding experienced by some users.
- If there are no contraindications, CHC can be used for 3 months either cyclically or continuously. Longer-term use is based on clinical judgement.

8.12.2 Missing threads
- If previously palpable threads become impalpable there are three main issues to consider:
  o the threads may have been drawn up into the uterine cavity
  o the device may have been expelled
  o the device may have translocated into the abdominal cavity.
- If the threads cannot be felt, women are advised to use an alternative method of contraception until clinical assessment can be undertaken.
- At this assessment a pregnancy test is recommended.
  o The endocervical canal can be gently explored; however, an ultrasound scan to confirm the presence of the IUS within the uterine cavity is the preferred approach. Once correct placement has been determined the IUS can remain *in situ* or, if removal is required, an IUS thread retriever or forceps should be used.
  o If the ultrasound scan fails to locate the IUS then an abdominal X-ray is advised to exclude the presence of the device within the abdominal cavity before expulsion can be assumed.

8.12.3 Managing IUS insertion pain
- There is currently no evidence to support the routine use of NSAIDs for pain management during insertion; however, NSAIDs are effective in the management of post-insertion pain.

- The literature regarding use of intracervical anaesthesia currently suggests that neither topical nor intracervical local anaesthetic gel prior to IUS insertion decrease pain scores during insertion. Routine use of paracervical local anaesthetic blocks may cause slightly more pain, without any obvious additional benefit; they may be of benefit in those women who require cervical dilation or who are particularly anxious.
- There is currently no evidence to suggest a particular type of forceps is associated with reduced insertion pain.

8.12.4 Pregnancy associated with an IUS

- As amenorrhoea is common in IUS users, women with pregnancy symptoms should seek medical advice.
- The site of the pregnancy should be confirmed by ultrasound scan.
- Additionally, the presence of an IUS in the uterine cavity increases the risk of early or mid-trimester pregnancy loss, sepsis and pre-term labour.
- If a woman presents before 12 weeks of pregnancy the device should be removed if the threads are visible but the uterus should not be instrumented.
- If the pregnancy is greater than 12 weeks the IUS should be left *in situ*. It is normally expelled with the placenta at delivery. If the IUS is not found at delivery then an abdominal X-ray should be performed to exclude translocation.
- There is currently no evidence that the presence of an IUS during pregnancy is associated with birth defects.

8.12.5 Actinomycosis-like organisms

- Actinomycosis-like organisms are normal commensals of the genital tract and their presence is not diagnostic of a disease process.
- Symptoms of pelvic actinomycosis including pain, dyspareunia, excessive discharge, and an adnexal mass.
  - in the absence of symptoms it is not necessary to remove the IUC
  - if symptoms are present IUS removal should be considered followed by antibiotics in accordance with local policy.

8.12.6 Syncope and bradycardia at insertion

- Bradycardia is a heart rate of <60 beats per minute, although symptoms do not typically occur until the heart rate reaches <40 beats per minute.
- Symptoms include feeling faint, dizziness and light-headedness, pallor, sweating, nausea and vomiting, and loss of consciousness which may be associated with twitching or a brief seizure.
- If associated with IUS insertions the symptoms occur as a result of vagal stimulation following dilation of the internal cervical os or instrumentation of the uterus.
- Symptoms are generally transient and resolve as the bradycardia resolves.
- With regard to management, the procedure should be stopped and the foot of the examination couch raised. Pulse and blood pressure should be monitored and supplemental oxygen given at 10–15 L/min.

- If pulse is less than 40 beats per minute and the IUS is in the uterine cavity the device should be removed and atropine administered (500 mcg IV or IM into the mid thigh). If there is no improvement after 5 mins call for emergency assistance or an ambulance. A further dose of atropine can be given after 5 mins for IV and 10 mins for IM administration.

8.12.7 IUS perforation

- If recognized at the time of the IUS fit, removal should be undertaken.
- If IUS perforation is identified at a later date, surgical removal by laparoscopy is advised.

8.12.8 Failure to insert an IUS

- The procedure is abandoned, bridging contraception provided and a follow-up appointment scheduled with a more experienced fitter.

8.12.9 Suspected pelvic infection

- If pelvic infection is clinically diagnosed appropriate antibiotics are commenced, keeping the IUS *in situ*. Current recommendations for the treatment of PID are:
  - ceftriaxone 500 mg single dose followed by
    oral doxycycline 100 mg twice daily plus
    metronidazole 400 mg twice daily for 14 days, OR
  - oral ofloxacin 400 mg twice daily plus oral metronidazole 400 mg twice daily for 14 days; both regimens provide cover against chlamydia and gonorrhoea as well as aerobic and anaerobic organisms. See the British Association for Sexual Health and HIV (www.BASHH.org) for further details.
- Only remove the IUS if symptoms fail to improve following 72 hours of antibiotic use.
- Ensure partner notification and sexual health advice is undertaken.
- Advise the woman not to have sex until the infection has been treated and her partner has completed their course of appropriate antibiotics.

8.13 Myths and misconceptions

- **The IUS causes weight gain** – there is no evidence to suggest that the IUS causes additional weight gain. Unfortunately women gain weight over time.
- **The IUS reduces your sex drive** – there is no current evidence to support an association.
- **An IUS can only be used by women who have had children** – the IUS is suitable for all women of reproductive age whether they have had children or not.
- **Women who are taking anticoagulants cannot have an IUS fitted** – this is not true; in fact an IUS may reduce menstrual blood loss associated with the use of this medication.

> **EXAMPLE**
>
> **A 32 year old woman attends for an IUS fitting. She is in a new relationship and was therefore offered an STI screen prior to her IUS fit. She is positive for genital chlamydia but is asymptomatic. She wants the IUS to be fitted immediately.**
>
> *What do you do?*
>
> 1. Confirm infection is asymptomatic.
> 2. Following counselling about the possible risks, an IUS could be inserted in an asymptomatic woman who has completed antibiotic treatment or on the day that treatment is commenced.
> 3. If the results of an infection screen are not available at the time of IUS fitting, the IUS should still be inserted without antibiotic prophylaxis, providing the woman is asymptomatic, contactable and willing to return for treatment if necessary.
> 4. In women with symptoms of possible or confirmed infection, IUS insertion should be delayed until the infection is treated and symptoms have resolved and a bridging method provided.

References

British Association for Sexual Health and HIV (2011) *UK National Guideline for the Management of Pelvic Inflammatory Disease.* Clinical Effectiveness Group. [available at www.bashh.org – accessed April 2016]

British National Formulary, September 2014–March 2015.

FSRH (2013) *Service Standards for Resuscitation in Sexual and Reproductive Health Services.* [www.fsrh.org/documents/clinical-standards-resuscitation-jan2013/ – accessed June 2016]

FSRH (2015) *Intrauterine Contraception.* Clinical Effectiveness Unit. [www.fsrh.org/documents/cec-ceu-guidance-iuc-apr-2015/ – accessed June 2016]

Heinemann, K. *et al.* (2015a) Risk of uterine perforation with levonorgestrel-releasing and copper intrauterine devices in the European Active Surveillance Study on Intrauterine Devices. *Contraception,* **91**: 274–279.

Heinemann, K. *et al.* (2015b) Comparative contraceptive effectiveness of levonorgestrel-releasing and copper intrauterine devices: the European Active Surveillance Study for Intrauterine Devices. *Contraception,* **91**: 280–283.

Office for National Statistics (2009) Opinions Survey Report No. 41 *Contraception and Sexual Health,* 2008/09.

UKMEC (2016) *UK Medical Eligibility Criteria for Contraceptive Use* [www.fsrh.org/standards-and-guidance/uk-medical-eligibility-criteria-for-contraceptive-use/ – accessed June 2016]

Chapter 9
Copper intrauterine devices

Over 180 million women worldwide use IUDs, with nearly 50% of these users in China. In the UK, only 6% of women use this form of contraception, probably because of concerns and myths attached to this method. The available IUDs in the UK are small copper-containing devices with most having a central frame made of polyethylene impregnated with barium sulphate to make them radiopaque. They come in varying shapes and sizes, including a frameless device called a GyneFix. Most devices contain more than 300 mm² of copper, making them a highly effective, reversible, inexpensive contraceptive option for women.

9.1 Potential users

9.1.1 Most appropriate users

- IUDs are an ideal choice for women who request a reliable non-hormonal method of contraception.
- The IUD is suitable for women until contraception is no longer required, providing there are no contraindications (see *Appendix*).
- An IUD can be used in women who have not had a previous pregnancy and continuation rates are similar for parous and nulliparous women.
- As the IUD provides immediately reversible contraception it is well suited to women wishing to space pregnancies.
- An IUD offers long-term effective contraception and so it provides a suitable alternative to sterilization for women who have completed their families.
- An IUD may be used as a method of emergency contraception (see *Chapter 13*).
- An IUD can be used for women with undetectable β-hCG and a history of trophoblastic disease.

9.1.2 Not suitable for the following users

The IUD is not suitable for women (for further information look at UKMEC in *Appendix*):

- with unexplained vaginal bleeding
- with post-partum and post-abortion sepsis
- post-partum between 48 hours and 4 weeks post-delivery
- with persistently elevated β-hCG or malignant disease
- with cervical cancer awaiting treatment
- with endometrial cancer
- with current pelvic inflammatory disease
- with current chlamydia or gonorrhoea (unless the infection is asymptomatic and treatment is given. Decision whether or not to fit should be made on a case-by-case basis)
- with known pelvic tuberculosis
- with known serious cardiac conditions or arrhythmias where a vasovagal collapse may have serious consequences
- HIV positive with a CD4 count <200 cells/mm^3.

9.2 Available IUDs in the UK

Details of the range of IUDs available in the UK are provided in *Table 9.1.*

Table 9.1. IUDs available in the UK

Trade name	Copper content	Location of copper	Cavity length	Duration of use	Cost
Ancora 375 Ag	375 mm²	Vertical stem	>6.5 cm	5 years	£9.95
Ancora 375 Cu	375 mm²	Vertical stem	>6.5 cm	5 years	£7.95
Copper T 380A	380 mm²	Vertical stem and copper sleeve on each arm	6–9 cm	10 years	£8.95
Cu-Safe T300	300 mm²	Vertical stem	>5 cm	5 years	£9.11
Flexi-T 300	300 mm²	Vertical stem	>5 cm	5 years	£9.47
Flexi-T + 380	380 mm²	Vertical stem and copper sleeve on each arm	>6 cm	5 years	£10.06
GyneFix	330 mm²	6 copper sleeves on polypropylene thread	Any size	5 years	£27.11
Load 375	375 mm²	Vertical stem	>7 cm	5 years	£8.52
Mini TT 380 Slimline	380 mm²	Vertical stem and copper sleeves fitted flush on to distal portion of each horizontal arm	>5 cm	5 years	£12.46
Multiload Cu375	375 mm²	Vertical stem	6–9 cm	5 years	£9.24
Multi-Safe 375	375 mm²	Vertical stem	6–9 cm	5 years	£8.96
Multi-Safe 375 Short Stem	375 mm²	Vertical stem	5–7 cm	5 years	£8.80

Trade name	Copper content	Location of copper	Cavity length	Duration of use	Cost
Neo-Safe T380	380 mm²	Vertical stem	6.5–9 cm	5 years	£13.31
Novaplus T 380 Ag	380 mm²	Vertical stem	Mini is 5 cm and normal size is 6.5–9 cm	5 years	£12.50
Novaplus T 380 Cu	380 mm²	Vertical stem	Mini is 5 cm and normal size is 6.5–9 cm	5 years	£10.95
Nova-T 380	380 mm²	Vertical stem	6.5–9 cm	5 years	£15.20
T-Safe 380A QuickLoad	380 mm²	Vertical stem with copper collar on the distal portion of each arm	6.5–9 cm	10 years	£10.47 for capsule load or £10.25 for QuickLoad
TT 380 Slimline	380 mm²	Vertical stem, and copper sleeves fitted flush on to distal portion of each horizontal arm	6.5–9 cm	10 years	£12.46
UT 380 Short	380 mm²	Vertical stem	5–7 cm	5 years	£11.22
UT 380 Standard	380 mm²	Vertical stem	6.5–9 cm	5 years	£11.22

Data from *British National Formulary* 2015.

9.3 Mechanism of action

- The main mechanism of action is to prevent fertilization through a foreign body effect and the copper ion's toxicity to sperm and ova.
- All IUDs increase the number of leukocytes in the endometrium. This produces a 'sterile' inflammatory endometrial response helping to prevent implantation. This reaction is enhanced by copper. Copper also affects endothelial enzymes, glycogen metabolism and oestrogen uptake.
- Copper content of the cervico-uterine mucus is high and this inhibits sperm penetration.
- An IUD is not an abortifacient because medicolegally, pregnancy begins at implantation not fertilization.

9.4 Efficacy

- Overall this method is associated with a failure rate of around 2% after 10 years and 0.1–1% after the first year of use. This equates to a failure rate of up to 2 in 1000 over 5 years.
- FSRH (2015) recommend the use of T-shaped IUDs containing 380 mm² of copper with banded copper on the arms of the device.

9.5 Pros and cons of IUDs

9.5.1 Advantages

- Long-term (up to 10 years depending on the device fitted), highly effective contraception, with no delay in return to fertility following removal.
- Non-hormonal contraceptive method, therefore no hormonal side-effects.
- Effective immediately after fitting.
- Non-intercourse related method of contraception.
- No drug interactions.
- Can be used when breast-feeding.
- Very low morbidity, with a mortality rate of less than 1 per 500 000 users.
- The most effective method of emergency contraception:
  - can be fitted up to 5 days after unprotected sexual intercourse at any time in the cycle
  - can also be fitted up to 5 days following the earliest estimated time of ovulation, even if multiple episodes of unprotected sex have occurred.
- High acceptability with first year continuation rates of almost 80%. IUDs are ideal for nulliparous women and those spacing their children or for those whose family is complete.
- Inexpensive and very cost-effective contraceptive method.
- Highly effective method of contraception.
- May give up to 50% protection against the development of endometrial cancer.

9.5.2 Disadvantages

- May cause menstrual irregularities, with intermenstrual bleeding and spotting occurring more commonly within the first 6 months after IUD insertion.
- Pain or discomfort may be experienced for a few hours to several days following insertion.
- Failure to fit the IUD correctly – although uncommon, failure may occur as a result of pain during insertion, anxiety or difficulties passing the uterine sound or device through the cervix; this may be due to anatomical anomaly or operator technique. The woman should be offered an alternative appointment with another more experienced fitter, with care taken to provide an alternative method of contraception in the interim.
- Periods may become heavier, more prolonged and painful. Periods may last 1–2 days longer, with blood loss increasing by about one-third. There may be more pre-/post-menstrual spotting and dysmenorrhoea. Intermenstrual bleeding and spotting is common in the first 3–6 months of IUD use. About 10% of women will discontinue using an IUD in the first year citing menstrual bleeding +/− pain as the main reason for removal. These problems may be managed with NSAID medication.
- IUDs provide no protection against STIs.
- About 1 in 20 IUDs are expelled, with this more likely to occur within the first 3 months of fitting, and the rate is similar for all types. This can lead to an unplanned pregnancy.

- Risk of pelvic infection is associated with IUD insertion and is increased 6-fold within the first 20 days following IUD insertion (1.6 per 1000 women-years). After day 20 the infection risk is low and remains low. The overall risk of PID is <1 in 100 in low-risk women.
- Uterine perforation is an uncommon event and may occur in up to 2 per 1000 insertions. Different IUDs are not associated with an increased or decreased risk of perforation, but the risk is increased in women who are breast-feeding. Perforation rates are influenced by fitter experience and the risk is higher in first-time users compared to previous users.
- IUDs are associated with a low risk of pregnancy. However, if pregnancy does occur approximately 15% will be ectopic. The incidence of ectopic pregnancy in IUD users is 0.08 per 100 women-years compared to 1.1 per 100 in UK women not using any contraception each year. Therefore, while the absolute risk of an ectopic pregnancy is lower in users of IUDs when compared to a background population, if a pregnancy does occur approximately 1 in 6 will be ectopic.

9.6 Counselling

- A relevant medical history to ensure medical eligibility, along with comprehensive counselling encompassing the advantages, disadvantages, side-effects (including perforation and expulsion rates), fitting procedure, and when to seek advice is advisable prior to the fitting of an IUD.
- Effective counselling helps ensure patient satisfaction and longevity of method use.
- STI history and screen (chlamydia screening as a minimum) is recommended prior to IUD insertion in women under 25 years old, or in women older than 25 with a new partner or more than 1 partner in the preceding 12 months. In asymptomatic women attending for insertion of an IUD there is no need to delay the fitting until results of a screen are available, providing that a screen has been or is taken at the time of fitting and the woman will return for treatment if required. If the IUD is fitted as an emergency, prophylactic treatment for chlamydia +/− gonorrhoea may be considered for women who are symptomatic or at high risk of infection.
- There is no need to routinely screen for bacterial vaginosis or candida infection.
- Pregnancy should be excluded prior to IUD insertion. Therefore, advise no sex following their period or provide a bridging method or fit as emergency contraception (see *Chapter 13*).
- Advise women to seek help immediately if they are concerned that they might be pregnant in order to perform a pregnancy test and, if positive, arrange an urgent ultrasound scan to locate the site of the pregnancy.
- Provide written information about the method, such as the Family Planning Association leaflet (available at www.fpa.org.uk). See *Table 9.2* for a summary of topics to be included during the discussion and in written information.

Table 9.2. Topics to include during counselling and in written information

Topics
Advantages and disadvantages
Efficacy and mechanism of action
Perforation rate – up to 2 per 1000; the rate is increased 6-fold in breast-feeding women less than 36 weeks since delivery (Heinemann *et al.*, 2015a)
Expulsion rate – 1 in 20, highest in the first 3 months post-insertion and during menstruation
Infection – 6-fold increased risk of PID in the first 20 days post-insertion, after which risk is low and remains low
Pregnancy and ectopic risk – pregnancy risk is 2 in 1000 over 5 years and ectopic risk was recently reported as 0.08 per 100 women-years (Heinemann *et al.*, 2015b)
Bleeding pattern – intermenstrual spotting is common for 3–6 months post-insertion; pre- and post-menstrual spotting is common and periods are often more painful
Contraception until fitting – abstain and continue current method of contraception

9.7 IUD starting regimen

This is described in *Table 9.3* below.

Table 9.3. Starting regimens for IUDs

Circumstances	Start when?	Extra precautions for seven days?
Menstruating	At any time in the cycle if reasonably certain the woman is not pregnant (avoiding insertion when menstrual flow is heavy thereby reducing subsequent expulsion)	No
Amenorrhoeic	Any time if reasonably certain the woman is not pregnant	No
Post-abortion or miscarriage (<24 weeks of gestation)	Immediately	No
	At any time by an experienced clinician as long as there is no concern that the pregnancy is ongoing	No
Post-partum: breast-feeding or bottle feeding	Immediately postpartum (<48 hours) or after day 28 (including following a Caesarean section) as long as she is not pregnant	No
Switching from other hormonal methods	Immediate start as long as the previous method has been used correctly and consistently	No
Switching from a non-hormonal method	Immediate start as long as the previous method has been used correctly and consistently	No

9.8 IUD insertion

- Undertake a bimanual examination to assess the size, position, shape and motility of the uterus and to exclude pathology.

- Using a non-touch (aseptic) technique insert a speculum and then apply forceps (Allis or tenaculum) to the cervix to stabilize it and reduce the risk of perforation.
- Assess cavity length with a uterine sound.
- Insert the IUD as per the product recommendations, ensuring that framed devices are placed at the fundus.
- Trim the threads to approximately 3 cm long.

9.9 Post IUD insertion advice

- Rest for a few minutes following the fitting.
- Instructions should be given on how and when to check IUD threads and when to seek advice; for example, if the threads feel longer than normal, if the woman is unable to feel the threads, or if the tip of the device is felt.
- Post-insertion pain is common in the first few days up to a week after insertion; however, if this is not resolved with simple analgesics individuals are advised to return for assessment.
- If there are symptoms suggestive of infection, such as foul-smelling discharge, abdominal pain and fever, medical advice and assessment is recommended.

9.10 Routine follow-up

- A 6 week follow-up appointment for assessment of bleeding, infection, expulsion and perforation is routinely undertaken. During this consultation women are routinely asked about bleeding and if any pain has been experienced. In addition, determine if the IUD threads have been felt and if there are any problems with sex (can the threads be felt during sex and if so do they need shortening?). The woman is examined to check thread length, ensure that the IUD stem cannot be felt in the cervical canal and that cervical excitation is not present.
- Routine yearly medical checks are not required. Women should be advised to return if they are unable to feel the IUD threads, have unexplained abdominal pain or have missed a period or have unscheduled bleeding after the first 3–6 months.

9.11 Return to fertility and device removal

- When an IUD is removed there is no delay in return to fertility because the hormonal cycle is not altered.
- The device can be removed at any time in the cycle. If the woman does not wish to become pregnant then she should be advised to use condoms for the 7 days preceding removal.

9.12 Managing side-effects and complications

9.12.1 Spotting or bleeding

- Spotting or light bleeding is commonly experienced during the first 3–6 months of IUD use, but it usually decreases with time.

- If bleeding continues or is heavy and prolonged a careful history and examination should be undertaken, plus additional investigations to exclude STIs, pregnancy and gynaecological pathology, as appropriate.
- An antifibrinolytic such as tranexamic acid 1 g taken 3 times a day can be taken on days 1–4 of bleeding +/– an NSAID (ibuprofen 400 mg 3 times a day or mefenamic acid 500 mg 3 times a day).
- If heavy bleeding is unacceptable or causes anaemia, discuss changing the contraceptive method to an IUS or an alternative LARC.

9.12.2 Vaginal discharge

- An increased watery or mucoid discharge is common; if this becomes profuse, persistent or offensive it is important to rule out infection.
- Bacterial vaginosis has been found in some studies to be more common among IUD users than among non-IUD users. However, recent studies indicate that it is the irregular bleeding rather than the presence of the IUD that is associated with bacterial vaginosis.

9.12.3 Missing threads

- If previously palpable threads become impalpable there are three main issues to consider:
  - the threads may have been drawn up into the uterine cavity
  - the device has been expelled
  - the device has translocated into the abdominal cavity.
- If the threads cannot be felt, women are advised to use an alternative method of contraception until clinical assessment can be undertaken.
- At this assessment a pregnancy test is recommended.
  - The endocervical canal can be gently explored; however, an ultrasound scan to confirm the presence of the IUD within the uterine cavity is the preferred approach. Once correct placement has been determined, the IUD can remain *in situ* or, if removal is required, an IUD thread retriever or removal forceps should be used.
  - If the ultrasound scan fails to locate the IUD then an abdominal X-ray is advised to exclude the presence of the device within the abdominal cavity before expulsion can be assumed.

9.12.4 Managing IUD insertion pain

- There is currently no evidence to support the use of NSAIDs for pain management prior to IUD insertion; however, NSAIDs are effective in treating post-insertion pain.
- The literature regarding use of intracervical anaesthesia currently suggests that neither topical nor intracervical local anaesthetic gel prior to IUD insertion decrease pain scores during insertion. Routine use of paracervical local anaesthetic blocks may cause slightly more pain, without any obvious additional benefit; they may be of benefit in those women who require cervical dilation or who are anxious.
- There is currently no evidence to suggest a particular type of forceps is associated with reduced insertion pain.

9.12.5 Pregnancy with an IUD *in utero*

- Women should seek urgent advice if they have a late or missed period. An ectopic pregnancy should be ruled out by performing an ultrasound scan to confirm the location of the pregnancy.
- Additionally, the presence of an IUD in the uterine cavity increases the risk of early or mid-trimester pregnancy loss, sepsis and pre-term labour.
- If a woman presents before 12 weeks of pregnancy the device should be removed if the threads are visible but the uterus should not be instrumented.
- If the pregnancy is greater than 12 weeks the IUD should be left *in situ*. It is normally expelled with the placenta at delivery. If the IUD is not found at delivery then an abdominal X-ray should be performed to exclude translocation.

9.12.6 Actinomycosis-like organisms

- Actinomycosis-like organisms are common commensals of the genital tract and their presence is not diagnostic of a disease process.
- Symptoms of pelvic actinomycosis include pain, dyspareunia, excessive discharge, and an adnexal mass:
  - in the absence of symptoms it is not necessary to remove the IUD
  - if symptoms are present, IUD removal should be considered followed by antibiotics in accordance with local policy.

9.12.7 Syncope and bradycardia at IUD insertion

- Bradycardia is a heart rate of <60 beats per minute, although symptoms do not typically occur until the heart rate reaches <40 beats per minute.
- Symptoms include feeling faint, dizziness and light-headedness, pallor, sweating, nausea and vomiting, and loss of consciousness which may be associated with twitching or a brief seizure.
- If associated with IUD insertion the symptoms occur as a result of vagal stimulation following dilation of the internal cervical os or instrumentation of the uterus.
- Symptoms are generally transient and resolve as the bradycardia resolves.
- With regard to management, the procedure should be stopped and the foot of the examination couch raised. Pulse and blood pressure should be monitored and supplemental oxygen given at 10–15 L/min.
- If pulse is less than 40 beats per minute and the IUD is in the uterine cavity the device should be removed and atropine administered at 500 mcg IV or IM into the mid thigh. If there is no improvement after 5 mins, call for emergency assistance or an ambulance. A further dose of atropine can be given after 5 min for IV and 10 min for IM administration.

9.12.8 IUD perforation

- If recognized at the time of IUD fit, removal should be undertaken.
- If IUD perforation is identified at a later date, surgical removal by laparoscopy is advisable because copper IUDs can cause an inflammatory reaction within the peritoneal cavity, leading to adhesions.

9.12.9 Failure to insert an IUD

- The procedure is abandoned, bridging contraception provided and a follow-up appointment made to re-attempt insertion.
- A re-attempt could be scheduled towards the end of a woman's next period as the cervical os is slightly more open at this time.
- If re-attempt fails, either undertake a trial of insertion using a narrower device or refer to your local specialist.

9.12.10 Suspected pelvic infection

- If pelvic infection is clinically diagnosed, appropriate antibiotics are commenced with the IUD *in situ*. Current recommendations for the treatment of PID are:
  - ceftriaxone 500 mg single dose followed by
    oral doxycycline 100 mg twice daily plus
    metronidazole 400 mg twice daily for 14 days, OR
  - oral ofloxacin 400 mg twice daily plus oral metronidazole 400 mg twice daily for 14 days, both of which provide cover against chlamydia and gonorrhoea, as well as aerobic and anaerobic organisms. See the British Association for Sexual Health and HIV (www.BASHH.org) for further details.
- Only remove the IUD if symptoms fail to improve following 72 hours of antibiotic use.
- Ensure partner notification and sexual health advice is undertaken.
- Advise the woman not to have sex until the infection has been treated and her partner has completed their course of appropriate antibiotics.

9.13 Myths and misconceptions

- **IUDs cause infection** – this is not true. Unprotected sex with a partner infected with an STI causes pelvic infection. Women using a copper IUD have no protection against the upper genital tract sequelae of STIs.
- **An IUD will cause scarring of the Fallopian tubes and infertility** – previous use of an IUD in nulliparous women is not associated with tubal factor infertility; however, untreated chlamydial infection is.
- **Partners will be aware of the presence of the IUD during sexual intercourse and it will cause pain** – the IUD threads rarely cause discomfort and soften with ongoing use. The IUD will not be dislodged by sexual intercourse. There is no reason why an IUD should negatively affect sexual pleasure or cause pain or discomfort during sex.
- **Women who are at risk of infective endocarditis cannot have an IUD** – the presence of risk factors for endocarditis such as valvular heart disease or a previous history of endocarditis are not contraindications to IUD use and prophylactic antibiotics are not required for insertion or removal of IUDs.

EXAMPLE

A 28 year old with a 6 month history of irregular bleeding attends clinic requesting an IUD.

What questions do you ask? Would you insert an IUD?

1. History and nature of the bleeding.
2. Cervical screening history.
3. Past medical history.
4. STI risk assessment.
5. Examination of the cervix and STI screen, depending on the history.
6. Refer for assessment if bleeding continues and investigations are negative.
7. At present do not insert the IUD but offer an alternative until the bleeding is investigated.

References

British Association for Sexual Health and HIV (2011) *UK National Guideline for the Management of Pelvic Inflammatory Disease*. Clinical Effectiveness Group. [available at www.bashh.org – accessed April 2016]

British National Formulary, September 2014–March 2015.

FSRH (2013) *Service Standards for Resuscitation in Sexual and Reproductive Health Services*.
[www.fsrh.org/documents/clinical-standards-resuscitation-jan2013/ – accessed June 2016]

FSRH (2015) *Intrauterine Contraception*. Clinical Effectiveness Unit.
[www.fsrh.org/documents/cec-ceu-guidance-iuc-apr-2015/ – accessed June 2016]

Heinemann, K. *et al*. (2015a) Risk of uterine perforation with levonorgestrel-releasing and copper intrauterine devices in the European Active Surveillance Study on Intrauterine Devices. *Contraception*, **91**: 274–279.

Heinemann, K. *et al*. (2015b) Comparative contraceptive effectiveness of levonorgestrel-releasing and copper intrauterine devices: the European Active Surveillance Study for Intrauterine Devices. *Contraception*, **91**: 280–283.

Office for National Statistics (2009) Opinions Survey Report No. 41 *Contraception and Sexual Health*, 2008/09.

UKMEC (2016) *UK Medical Eligibility Criteria for Contraceptive Use*
[www.fsrh.org/standards-and-guidance/uk-medical-eligibility-criteria-for-contraceptive-use/ – accessed June 2016]

Chapter 10
Barrier methods

Barrier methods of contraception include male and female condoms, diaphragms and cervical caps. The male condom is used by 8% of couples globally and is the fourth most popular birth control method worldwide. In the UK, 25% of couples state that their main contraceptive method is the male condom and about 1% the female condom. Caps and diaphragms are used by less than 1% of couples.

- Male condoms fit over an erect penis and female condoms are worn in the vagina – both act as a barrier to sperm.
- Female condoms consist of a loose sheath with an inner ring at the closed end; this is placed in the vagina. The second ring on the rim of the sheath covers the vulva (*Figure 10.1*).
- A cervical cap or diaphragm covers the cervix and spermicide should be applied before insertion.

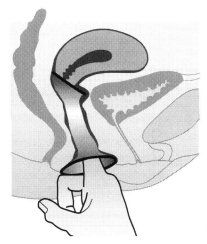

Figure 10.1. Positioning a female condom.

10.1 Potential users

10.1.1 Most appropriate users

- Male condoms can be used by almost everyone.
- Male and female condoms are not only a barrier method of contraception but also provide protection against STIs.
- Female condoms, diaphragms and cervical caps are most suitable for women who are comfortable with touching their genital area because they need to be inserted into the vagina.
- Barrier methods are ideal for couples spacing their family and in those where an unplanned pregnancy would be accepted.

10.1.2 Not suitable for the following users

- Couples wanting a highly effective contraceptive. They may wish to use an additional method.
- Male condoms may not be suitable for men with erectile dysfunction. Their partner may prefer to use another contraceptive method.
- Those with a true latex allergy. They could try male or female condoms made from polyurethane.
- Diaphragms and caps may not be suitable for those with:
  - a history of toxic shock syndrome
  - lax vaginal walls because the diaphragm or cap may move during sex and so not cover the cervix
  - an unusually shaped or positioned cervix because placement may be difficult
  - a sensitivity to spermicide
  - a sensitivity to latex; they may wish to try the Caya diaphragm which is made of silicone

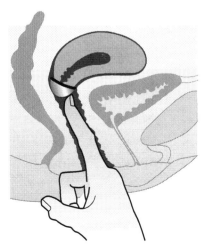

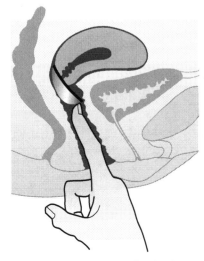

Figure 10.2. Placing a cervical cap. **Figure 10.3.** Insertion of a diaphragm.

○ recurrent urinary tract infections

○ recurrent vaginal infections

○ HIV – due to the risk associated with the spermicide rather than the diaphragm itself; nonoxynol-9 may increase the risk of HIV transmission

○ a recent pregnancy or second trimester abortion; women are advised to wait 6 weeks post-delivery before caps and diaphragms are sized and fitted.

10.2 Available barrier methods

10.2.1 Male condoms

- Male condoms are made from latex, polyurethane, synthetic polyisoprene, or deproteinized latex.
- Some condoms are pre-lubricated.
- There are a variety of sizes, flavours and shapes available.
- Some condoms fit an individual better than others and so there is an element of trial and error for each individual in finding the best option.
- Silicone-based pre-lubricated condoms are recommended. There is no evidence that condoms lubricated with spermicide (nonoxynol-9) provide additional contraceptive protection when compared with condoms lubricated with a non-spermicide. Nonoxynol-9 may also increase STI transmission as a result of its irritant effect.
- Male condoms reduce the risk of STI transmission when used for oral/anal as well as vaginal sex.

10.2.2 Female condoms

These are made of polyurethane and are usually pre-lubricated with a non-spermicidal lubricant.

10.2.3 Diaphragms and caps

Table 10.1 shows the range of diaphragms and caps available in the UK, including cost.

Table 10.1. Diaphragms and caps

	Presentation	Brand	Size	Cost
Diaphragm	Silicone – coiled spring	Milex, Omniflex	60–90 mm (in 5 mm increments	£9.31
	Silicone – arcing spring	Milex arcing style, Ortho all-flex	60–90 mm (in 5 mm increments)	£8.35
	Silicone – flexible rim	Caya	One size	£20.54* £31.50** £38.99***
Cap	Silicone	Femcap	22, 26, and 30 mm	£15.29 £39.99*

* For purchase by health care services direct from distributor [accessed April 2015]

** For personal purchase direct from distributor [April 2015]

***For personal purchase – prices checked on www.amazon.co.uk [April 2015].

Other data from *British National Formulary* 2014.

- Diaphragms lie diagonally between the posterior fornix and pubic bone.
- Flat spring diaphragms have been discontinued.
- Coiled spring diaphragms are flexible and may be more comfortable during sexual intercourse.
- Arcing spring diaphragms are useful for women with lax vaginal walls, a retroverted uterus or for women in whom assessment of the vaginal length or cervical position is difficult.
- Flexible rim diaphragms are a single size which is suitable for approximately 80% of women. It is recommended that women are assessed prior to use to ensure the diaphragm fits.

10.3 Efficacy

Table 10.2 shows the efficacy of each of the barrier methods.

Table 10.2. Percentage failure rate of each barrier method

Method	Percentage failure rate	
	Typical	Perfect
Female condom	21	5
Male condom	18	2
Diaphragm	12	6
Cervical cap	32 (parous) 16 (nulliparous)	20 (parous) 9 (nulliparous)

- An unplanned pregnancy may occur with use of male and female condoms if:
  - they are fitted after genital touching has occurred
  - there are tears in the condom
  - a male condom slips off or penetration occurs outside the outer ring of the female condom
- The efficacy of diaphragm and cap can be reduced if it is:
  - damaged, for example, if a tear or hole is present
  - the incorrect size and the cervix is not covered
  - used without a spermicide
  - inserted 3 or more hours (2 or more for Caya diaphragm) before sexual intercourse and additional spermicide is not used
  - removed too soon after sex, i.e. less than 6 hours
  - used for repeated episodes of sex without the application of additional spermicide
  - used with oil-based products which may damage the latex.

10.4 Mechanism of action

- Barrier methods stop sperm and ovum meeting. They provide a barrier to the ejaculate and pre-ejaculate and work by preventing fertilization.

10.5 Pros and cons of barrier methods

10.5.1 Advantages

- Only need to be used when having sex.
- Provide protection for both partners against STIs (condoms).
- Are a non-hormonal method.
- Have no serious side-effects.
- Condoms, diaphragms and caps are available in a variety of sizes.
- Male condoms are easily available.
- Non-latex barriers are available.
- A female condom can be inserted up to 8 hours before sex.
- Female condoms are less likely to tear than the male condom.
- Diaphragms and caps can be inserted several hours before intercourse so that spontaneity can be maintained.
- The woman can control the use of contraception.
- Barrier methods are not compromised by drug therapy (for example, liver enzyme inducing drugs).
- Male condom use increases human papillomavirus clearance and cervical intra-epithelial neoplasia regression.

10.5.2 Disadvantages

- Barrier methods require motivation with each sexual episode.
- Barrier use may interrupt sex including reapplication of spermicide.
- Barrier methods are less effective than hormonal or intrauterine contraceptives.
- Latex sensitivity may occur (rare).
- Male condoms must be worn before there is any intimate contact.
- Male condoms may break or slip off during sex.
- Male condoms must be removed from the penis before it becomes flaccid.
- When using female condoms the penis must be inserted through the outer ring and not between the condom and vagina.
- Female condoms can slip out or be pushed into the vagina.
- The inner ring of the female condom may cause discomfort during sex.
- Female condoms can be noisy during sex.
- Most diaphragms and caps require fitting by a healthcare professional.
- Women must be comfortable with self-examination in order to insert and remove female barrier methods.
- Diaphragms and caps cannot be used until 6 weeks post-partum or 6 weeks after a second trimester abortion.
- Diaphragm and cap sizing needs to be rechecked after weight gain or loss of 3 kg or more.
- Diaphragms and caps do not reduce the risk of transmission of STIs.
- Women may find diaphragms and caps messy and dislike the idea of leaving them in place for 6 hours after sex.

10.6 Practical aspects

10.6.1 Male condoms

- Ask patients to check the 'use by' date and safety markings (kite marks or CE mark) on the packet to ensure they meet appropriate recognized standards for strength and quality.
- They should carefully remove the condom from the packet to ensure it does not become damaged.
- A new condom should be used for each new episode of sexual intercourse.
- The closed end (teat) of the condom should be squeezed to expel any air.
- The condom is rolled down over an erect penis.
- It may be more comfortable for men with a foreskin to put the condom on after the foreskin is pulled back. This enables the foreskin to move more freely during sex and it reduces the risk of the condom slipping off or tearing.
- After ejaculation and before the penis become flaccid the penis is withdrawn from the vagina with the bottom of the condom held in place to reduce slippage.
- The condom is then removed and disposed of in the bin rather than down a toilet.

Potential problems with male condoms

- Potential users should be advised that latex condoms (but not polyurethane condoms) can be caused to break if oil-based lubricants, such as body oil or lotion, cooking oil, baby oil, suntan lotion or petroleum jelly, are used.
- Oil-based vaginal preparations can damage condoms and make these methods less effective, including:
  - Canesten pessaries and cream
  - Cyclogest
  - Dalacin cream
  - E45 and similar preparations
  - Ecostatin
  - Fungilin
  - Gyno-Daktarin
  - Gyno-Pevaryl/Monistat
  - Nizoral
  - Witepsol-based products
- For anal intercourse the use of a water-based lubricant is recommended as it reduces the risk of breakage by 18%.

10.6.2 Female condoms

- Ask patients to check the 'use by' date and safety marking on the packet.
- Carefully remove the condom from the packet to ensure it does not become damaged.
- The female condom can be inserted into the vagina any time before sex.
- To insert the condom the woman should find a position in which she feels comfortable, such as lying down, squatting or with one leg elevated on a chair.

- Holding the closed end of the condom the inner ring is squeezed between thumb and finger.
- The labia are parted and the condom, along with the inner ring, is inserted into the vagina.
- The female condom should be pushed up into the vagina as far as possible.
- A tip to achieve correct placement is to put the index or middle finger (or both) into the open end of the condom until the inner ring is felt.
- The condom is then pushed so that the inner ring lies just above the pubic bone.
- The outer ring of the condom remains outside the vagina and lies up across the vulva.
- During sex the penis should be guided into the vagina through the centre of the outer ring of the condom.
- After sex the penis is withdrawn and the outer ring of the condom held in place.
- The condom is removed by twisting the outer ring to ensure the semen remains within the condom, then pulling the condom out and disposing of it in the bin.

10.6.3 Diaphragms

Each diaphragm comes with its own instructions but several general principles apply and are described below.
- The woman is examined and the correct size of diaphragm chosen; the size of the diaphragm equates to the approximate distance from the posterior fornix to the pelvic arch of the pubic bone and the largest size which feels comfortable, is ideal.
- The user is taught how to insert and remove the diaphragm (see below and *Figure 10.3*).
- Another method such as a condom should be used until the woman is confident inserting the device.
- A review 1–2 weeks after the initial assessment is advised to ascertain if the woman is comfortable using the method and if there are any problems. In addition, review of the diaphragm's position after insertion by the individual is recommended. Further checks are recommended:
  ○ if 3 kg of weight is lost or gained
  ○ following childbirth, miscarriage or abortion, because vaginal/cervical size and shape can change.
- Before sex the diaphragm should be checked to make sure there are no holes or tears. If it is out of shape it can be squeezed back into a circular shape.
- Approximately two 2 cm strips of spermicide (or 4 ml/1 teaspoon of acid-buffering lubricant for Caya) is applied to the upper surface of the diaphragm. For ease of insertion a small amount of spermicide can also be applied to the rim.
- With the index finger on the top of the diaphragm the two sides of the diaphragm are squeezed together. The diaphragm is inserted into the vagina in either a standing, squatting or lying position. It is pushed upwards and backwards so it covers the cervix.
- If sex occurs either after the diaphragm or cap has been in place for more than 3 hours or if sex is repeated with the device in place, additional spermicide is required by placing a full applicator of spermicidal cream into the vagina.
- The diaphragm is removed by hooking a finger under the diaphragm rim or loop. This is then pulled downwards.

- The diaphragm must be left in place for at least 6 hours after sex but no longer than 30 hours for latex diaphragms (24 hours for Caya).
- Once the diaphragm is removed it can be washed with warm water and mild soap. It is then rinsed, dried and stored in a cool dry place.

10.6.4 Caps

There are several caps available but the following general principles apply.
- Before use an individual is fitted with the correct size of cap and taught how to insert and remove it (see *Figure 10.2*).
- Ideally the cervix should be assessed and caps fitted mid-cycle.
- It is advisable that until an individual is comfortable using the device another method such as a condom is also used.
- One to two weeks after the initial assessment a review appointment is recommended to ascertain if the individual is comfortable using the method and if there are any problems with cap placement.
- A recheck is recommended following a pregnancy (similar to diaphragm users)
- Every time the cap is used:
  - it should be checked for damage
  - one-quarter of a teaspoon of spermicide is put in the dome and then some is spread around the rim, then the cap is flipped over and spermicide placed in the groove between the rim and the dome (see *Figure 10.4*).

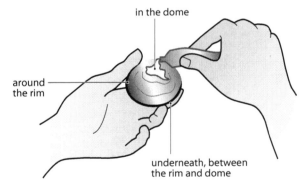

in the dome

around the rim

underneath, between the rim and dome

Figure 10.4. Use of spermicide with the cap. Remind the woman that if she is going to have sex more than once, more spermicide must be used and the position of the cap should be checked.

- To insert the cap the woman squeezes the sides together and inserts it into the vagina and over the cervix. The cap needs to fit well over the cervix and suction holds the cap in place.
- Before use the woman should check the cervix is covered by the cap.
- The cap must be left in place for at least 6 hours after sex, but for no longer than 48 hours.
- Once the cap is removed it can be washed with warm water and mild soap, rinsed and dried and then stored in a cool dry place.

Potential problems with diaphragms and caps

- The use of diaphragms and caps during menses is not recommended due to the potential risk of toxic shock syndrome.
- A repeat assessment of diaphragm/cap size is advised if the user gains or loses 3 kg in weight.
- If there is difficulty with insertion of the diaphragm the size should be reassessed and if necessary a smaller size chosen. An alternative option would be to try an arcing spring diaphragm.
- Women who suffer from recurrent UTIs when using a diaphragm should be advised to empty their bladder before and after sex. A smaller sized flat spring diaphragm or coil spring diaphragm could be tried. Alternatively she could change to using a cervical cap.
- In women complaining of vaginal soreness:
  - the size of diaphragm should be checked
  - investigate and treat any infection
  - consider a latex allergy
  - consider using Caya diaphragm and Caya diaphragm gel (non-spermicidal gel containing lactic acid).
- If the partner can feel the diaphragm the healthcare professional should:
  - check that the correct size is being used and that the cervix is covered
  - consider changing to coil spring or arcing diaphragm, or a cervical cap.

10.7 Myths and misconceptions

- **Discolouration of the diaphragm means it needs to be replaced** – this is incorrect; discolouration is normal but the functionality of the device is unaffected. Holes and tears, however, do affect the efficacy of the diaphragm and if either are found it should be replaced.
- **Both partners will be able to feel the diaphragm or cap during sex** – this is incorrect; if the correct size is used and the device is inserted correctly neither partner should be able to feel the diaphragm or cap. If the diaphragm or cap can be felt or is uncomfortable, a refit is recommended, and if the problem continues an alternative cap or diaphragm or alternative method of contraception could be tried.
- **A condom will not roll all the way to the end of the penis and so all condoms are too small** – this is incorrect; the most likely explanation is that the condom is inside out and so it should be removed and a new one tried.
- **Using two condoms provides increased protection** – this is not only incorrect but actually increases the chances of a failure, as friction between the condoms raises the likelihood of them both tearing. In addition a male and female condom should not be used at the same time. Furthermore, lubricant should not be applied inside a condom (gel-charging) as this can result in the condom slipping off.
- **Condoms cause premature ejaculation** – this is incorrect; a male condom does not cause premature ejaculation. In fact, wearing a condom may reduce sensation and be helpful. Furthermore, some condoms contain a small amount of lidocaine gel to help prevent premature ejaculation.

EXAMPLE

A 26 year old women presents with genital irritation which she suspects is due to her partner's condom.

What would your management plan be?

1. Confirm that the irritation is due to condom use – consider differential diagnoses such as a dermatological condition, for example, eczema or dermatitis.
2. Determine the type of condom used; is it lubricated with a spermicide? Reactions to spermicides are more common than latex allergy.
3. Advise changing to polyurethane or deproteinized latex condoms or consider using a diaphragm or cap.
4. Most cases of latex allergy are mild with reactions occurring 24–48 hours following exposure and limited to the site of contact. Very rarely, symptoms become generalized. Repeated exposure may increase the risk of a reaction occurring.
5. Occasionally further investigation is warranted with skin testing for the presence of immunoglobulin E antibodies against latex.

References

British National Formulary, September 2014–March 2015.

FSRH (2012) *Barrier Methods for Contraception and STI Prevention*. Clinical Effectiveness Unit.
[www.fsrh.org/documents/ceuguidancebarriermethodscontraceptionsdi/ – accessed June 2016]

Chapter 11
Fertility awareness

Fertility awareness is the generic term for what is colloquially known as the 'rhythm method' or 'using the safe period'. Using signs of the fertile phase of the menstrual cycle, pregnancies can be planned and also potentially avoided without the use of additional hormones or devices.

In the UK about 2% of couples use fertility awareness as their method of contraception, but worldwide many more use these methods to space their families. Natural family planning is effective if couples abstain from penetrative sex or use barrier methods during the fertile phase of the menstrual cycle.

'Withdrawal' (removing the penis from the vagina before ejaculation) is used by 4% of British couples as their method of contraception. This is seen by many to be a 'natural' method and will be discussed in more detail at the end of the chapter.

11.1 Potential users

11.1.1 Most appropriate users

- Couples wanting to use a natural contraceptive method with no hormones or interruption of sex.
- Women using fertility awareness should have a regular menstrual cycle.
- Couples using fertility awareness are required to keep a diary, recognize the signs of the fertile phase and understand the importance of abstaining from sex or using barrier methods during this phase.
- Couples need to be highly motivated.
- These methods are ideal for couples who want to space their children and where an unplanned pregnancy would be accepted.

11.1.2 Not suitable for the following users

- Those wanting a highly effective method of contraception.
- Women who are taking teratogenic drugs.
- Women for whom pregnancy would put them at high risk of serious morbidity or mortality.
- Women with irregular menstrual cycles.
- Women who are post-partum and not breast-feeding.
- Women who are peri-menopausal.
- Women who have recently discontinued a hormonal contraceptive method. They should only rely on data once periods have returned and they have had a minimum of three regular cycles.
- Fertility awareness is not suitable for women who find it difficult to follow the instructions for recognizing the fertile phase or could not abstain or use barrier methods during this time.
- Withdrawal is not suitable for men:
  - who could not recognize the pre-ejaculatory phase
  - who may not comply on all occasions.

11.2 Available fertility awareness methods

These are summarized in *Table 11.1*.

Table 11.1. Fertility awareness methods in common use

Method	How it is used	What is required	How much does it cost?
Temperature	The basal body temperature is measured each morning before getting up	A sensitive digital thermometer	About £4
Calendar	This is recorded over a 12 month period to calculate the longest and shortest cycles	Calendar downloaded from www.fertilityuk.org/	No cost
Cervical mucus	Changes during the month are noted	Correct technique	No cost
Two day method	Avoid having sex if cervical secretions are noted on the day of observation and the day before	Correct technique	No cost
Symptothermal method (using a combination of methods)	Different fertility indicators are used; normally the menstrual calendar, body temperature and cervical mucus	Correct technique and documentation (fertility awareness calendar) plus thermometer	About £4
Lactational amenorrhoea method (LAM)	When a woman is fully breast-feeding within 6 months of the baby's birth	Correct technique	No cost
Devices for detecting fertile phase	Devices such as Persona detect the fertile phase by measuring urinary estriol-3-glucuronide and LH	Persona device	About £53

Costs checked March 2015 on www.amazon.co.uk.

11.3 Mechanism of action

Sperm survive up to 7 days in the cervical mucus during the fertile phase and an ovum will be receptive to fertilization for 24 hours. Therefore the fertile phase is thought to last up to 9 days (see *Figure 11.1*). Any method that can detect this fertile phase so that couples can either abstain or use a barrier method during this time may help prevent a pregnancy.

The withdrawal method requires a man to remove his penis from the vagina before he ejaculates.

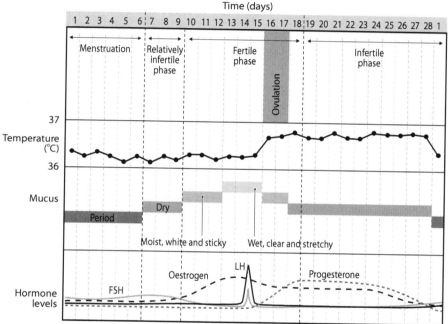

Figure 11.1. Signs used for fertility awareness methods when using the symptothermal method (a combination of the calendar method, basal body temperature and cervical secretions).

11.4 Efficacy

- The fertile window can vary from month to month. Therefore couples are required to avoid sex or use barrier methods for 8–9 days each month, even if they are using a number of fertile phase indicators.
- The failure rate using one indicator can be as high at 24%, but as low as 0.4% when using the symptothermal method (a combination of the calendar method, basal body temperature and cervical secretions).
- Devices such as Persona detect the fertile phase, giving a failure rate of 6% when used perfectly.
- Withdrawal has a failure rate of 4% with perfect use and 22% in typical use because the pre-ejaculate has been shown to contain motile sperm in many men.

11.5 Pros and cons of fertility awareness

11.5.1 Advantages

- Can be used to plan pregnancy as well as prevent conception.
- No known physical side-effects.
- Non-intercourse related method.
- No mechanical devices or hormones used.
- Acceptable to all cultures and religions.
- Once learnt by the user no further follow-up is necessary.

11.5.2 Disadvantages

- Has a relatively high failure rate in practice when using only one fertility awareness indicator.
- Requires commitment from both partners.
- Illness may affect body temperature readings.
- Successful use depends on education.
- Requires careful observation and record keeping, which may take time to learn.
- Users must have high motivation, requiring long periods of abstinence from intercourse or use of barrier methods.
- Does not protect against sexually transmitted infections.
- Does not offer the advantages of hormonal methods in reducing menstrual loss and dysmenorrhoea or endometrial/ovarian cancer.

11.6 Using the different methods

11.6.1 Temperature

- Once ovulation has occurred, progesterone is produced by the corpus luteum; this causes the basal body temperature to rise.
- Using a sensitive digital thermometer the woman takes her temperature before getting up and following at least 3 hours of rest.
- The post-ovulatory infertile phase can be detected by measuring a rise of 0.2°C on three consecutive days when compared to the previous six days.
- No additional method of contraception is needed once the post-ovulatory infertile phase has been identified until the start of menstruation.
- Using this method alone couples will need to avoid sex or use barrier methods for about 16 days each month (days 3 to 19 in a typical 28 day cycle): this is during the whole of the pre-ovulatory phase and will continue until the post-ovulation infertile phase begins.

11.6.2 Calendar method

- Normally 12 months of menstrual cycle data should be documented to accurately predict the fertile phase each month.

- The fertile phase when using the calendar method only normally lasts up to 16 days and abstinence or use of an additional method is required during this time (days 8 to 19 on a 28 day cycle).
- The shortest and longest cycle should be used to calculate the fertile period.
- The first fertile day is determined by subtracting 20 days from the shortest cycle.
- The last fertile day is established by subtracting 10 days from the longest cycle.
- The fertile phase should be constantly adjusted using data from the last 12 months.
- The simplified calendar method is a simpler method for those women with regular cycles between 26 and 32 days (see *Figure 11.2*).

Simplified calendar method

Women should have cycles between 26 and 32 days (no irregular cycles)
The first fertile day will always be day 8
The last fertile day will be day 19
Abstinence or barrier methods are required between day 8 and day 19 each month

---

Figure 11.2. Simplified calendar method.

11.6.3 Changes in cervical secretions and cervix

- During the ovulatory phase of the cycle women produce more oestradiol from the developing ovarian follicle which results in cervical secretions becoming abundant, stretchy and similar to raw egg white mid-cycle.
- Women need to record when they first notice any secretion and this is the start of the fertile phase. They then need to abstain or use a barrier method.
- Once the secretions have reached their peak day, where they will be similar to raw egg white, the secretions then become thicker and less abundant under the influence of progesterone. When this change has been present for a full 3 days the fertile phase ends and no additional method is required.
- Changes to the cervix may also indicate the fertile phase but should only be used in conjunction with other indicators.
- When the cervix feels high, soft and open, sex should be avoided or barrier methods used.
- No additional methods are needed when the cervix is low, firm and closed for consecutive 3 days.
- Use of barrier methods and spermicides may interfere with the use of cervical secretions as a fertile phase indicator. Other indicators, therefore, should also be used.

11.6.4 Two day method

- This is a modification of the cervical secretion method and is simple to learn.
- Secretions should be assessed in the late afternoon or evening.
- Abstinence or use of barriers is required when secretions are seen on the day of observation or the day before.
- Once there have been two consecutive dry days no additional methods are required.

11.6.5 Devices for detecting the fertile phase

- There are devices that detect the fertile phase by measuring urinary estriol-3-glucuronide and luteinizing hormone (LH).
- When increased levels of these hormones are measured, abstinence or additional barrier methods should be used.

11.6.6 Lactational amenorrhoea method (LAM)

Breast-feeding is a natural way to space children. Suckling suppresses LH and FSH, which results in amenorrhoea and stimulation of prolactin leading to lactation. LAM is very effective, offering 98% protection against pregnancy when the following conditions exist:

- A woman is fully or almost fully breast-feeding (feeding with no substitutes and at regular periods on demand, day and night)
- There are no long intervals between feeds, e.g. no more than 4 hours during the day and 6 hours during the night
- The baby is less than 6 months old
- Menstruation has not returned.

11.7 Withdrawal method

'Withdrawal' is the oldest method of birth control; it is still one of the most popular natural contraceptive methods worldwide. It can be practised by any couple at any time.

11.7.1 Advantages of withdrawal

- It is free of charge.
- It requires no prescription.
- It does not cause nausea or weight gain.
- It is acceptable to many users.

11.7.2 Disadvantages of withdrawal

- It has a high failure rate.
- Sex is often thought to be incomplete.
- It may be unsatisfying for both partners.
- Partial ejaculation of semen can occur resulting in failure of the method.
- It does not protect against STI/HIV transmission.

11.8 Myths and misconceptions

- **Fertility awareness is complicated and difficult to teach** – no it is not. Women with regular cycles who are motivated to use these methods can find all the necessary information on the internet. Instruction guides are available along with downloadable charts and a digital thermometer can be bought. Barrier methods are then used until a woman has enough data to accurately predict her fertile phase. See www.fertilityuk.org/ for further details.

- **Using fertility awareness as a contraceptive method results in a high risk of pregnancy** – this is not correct. Couples who consistently use several fertility indicators, such as with the symptothermal method, have a failure rate of just 0.4%.
- **Couples using withdrawal should be advised to use condoms to reduce their chance of an unplanned pregnancy** – there is no evidence to support this advice. Many couples are happy using withdrawal and often feel pressurized to change their method. The typical failure rates of withdrawal and condoms are similar, therefore couples should choose the method that most fits their needs.

EXAMPLE

A 28 year old woman is having problems working out her fertile phase using the calendar method. She has recorded her periods over the last 12 months with the shortest cycle from the first day of one period to the first day of the next being 24 days. Her longest cycle is 32 days.

What do you advise?

1. She can use the Standard days method to work out the first day of her fertile phase by taking 20 from her shortest cycle (24 days). Therefore her first fertile day is day 4 of each cycle.
2. Her last fertile day is calculated by subtracting 10 from her longest cycle (32 days). Therefore her last fertile day is day 22.
3. She would then have to abstain from sex or use an additional contraceptive method for 19 days each month.
4. To help shorten the fertile phase she may therefore use a second or even third indicator, such as using her basal body temperature or cervical secretions.

References

Office for National Statistics (2009) Opinions Survey Report No. 41 *Contraception and Sexual Health*, 2008/09.

FSRH (2015) *Fertility Awareness Methods*. Clinical Effectiveness Unit. [www.fsrh.org/documents/ceuguidancefertilityawarenessmethods/ – accessed June 2016]

Chapter 12
Male and female sterilization

Worldwide, sterilization is the most common method of contraception; female sterilization is used by 19% of women aged 15–49 who are married or in a relationship, and male sterilization is used by 2% of men worldwide. There are three methods of sterilization available in the UK: vasectomy for men and laparoscopic or hysteroscopic sterilization for women. Within England, there were just over 14 000 vasectomies performed in 2013. For female sterilization, about 9000 procedures were undertaken in 2013 in England.

12.1 Potential users

Sterilization is a permanent method of contraception suitable for all those who do not wish to have children or have completed their family.

12.1.1 Most appropriate users

Male and female sterilization can be used by the majority of men and women. It is most suitable for those who have completed their families and have had no surgery to the abdomen or testicles.

12.1.2 Not suitable for the following users

There are few conditions which would completely restrict an individual's eligibility to undergo sterilization; however, a delay may be recommended until the patient is medically fit for surgery or an experienced surgeon is available.

The procedure is normally conducted in a surgical day unit, but there may be certain circumstances which require extra preparation, precautions and counselling. For example:
- obesity (BMI >35) makes the procedure more difficult, and there is increased risk of wound infection and complications at time of surgery
- uterine fibroids may make it more difficult to localize the tubes
- large varicocele or hydrocele may make localizing the vas deferens more difficult.

For certain medical conditions, or following a related procedure, it may be more prudent to delay the procedure until the condition is evaluated, treated and/or changes or resolves. For example:

- post-abortion – it is advisable to delay sterilization until 6 weeks post-abortion, with the provision of alternative contraception
- current infection – it is advisable to allow time for effective treatment of the infection, be that pelvic inflammatory disease, epididymitis or sexually transmitted infection, or gastrointestinal or respiratory infection.

For other conditions it may be advisable that the procedure should be undertaken in a setting with an experienced surgeon and staff, equipment needed to provide general anaesthesia, and other back-up medical support. For these conditions, the capacity to decide on the most appropriate procedure and anaesthesia method is also needed. Alternative temporary methods of contraception should be provided, if referral is required or there is otherwise any delay. For example:

- a fixed uterus due to previous surgery or infection – the risk of laparotomy is increased and complications are more likely.

For hysteroscopic sterilization, immune suppression (e.g. corticosteroids) is a relative contraindication because it is probable that immunosuppressive therapy will negatively affect tissue response to the micro-inserts.

The manufacturers advise against performing an endometrial ablation at the time of fitting of these micro-inserts. Hysteroscopic sterilization should only be performed in women following an endometrial ablation if their tubal ostia are easily seen.

Endometrial ablation and other hysteroscopic procedures may result in displacement or removal of these micro-inserts, therefore it is advisable to check their location following such procedures using a recognized confirmation test.

12.2 Available methods of sterilization

These are summarized in *Table 12.1*.

Table 12.1. Summary of methods of sterilization

Method	Typical anaesthetic requirement	Time from procedure until current or additional contraception can be stopped
Vasectomy	Local	Once semen sample is negative for sperm – typically tested 12 weeks post-vasectomy
Laparoscopic tubal occlusion	General or regional – usually as a day case	Immediately effective so long as there are no viable sperm in the genital tract – contraception should be continued for at least a week
Hysteroscopic sterilization	None or local	3 months following transvaginal ultrasound scan or X-ray as first line or, alternatively, use hysterosalpingogram to confirm correct placement or blockage

12.3 Mechanism of action

- Sterilization interrupts or occludes the passage of sperm or ovum.

12.4 Pros and cons of sterilization

12.4.1 Advantages

- Non-hormonal method.
- Removes the need for future/on-going contraception.
- No hormonal side-effects.
- Rarely has a long-term effect on health.
- No effect on libido or sexual function.

12.4.2 Disadvantages

- A surgical procedure is required.
- Uncommonly, the vas deferens or Fallopian tube(s) may re-join, returning an individual to fertility, and so possibly leading to an unplanned pregnancy.
- Sterilization cannot be easily reversed and reversal is not available on the NHS.
- Sterilization does not protect against STIs.
- It takes up to 3 months for sterilization to be effective, depending on the method.
- Each method is associated with potential complications.
- There may be regret associated with the permanence of the procedure, particularly if circumstances change.

12.5 Counselling and consent

Discussion prior to sterilization is ideally undertaken with both partners present and encompasses the following:

- Ensuring that both partners do not want children, or if they already have children that their family is complete. Enquire about number of children, if they have family with their current partner, and if there are any circumstances in which they may wish to have a future pregnancy.
- Identify reasons for the sterilization to ensure that the method is appropriate and that there is no coercion on the part of the partner.
- Ask about past medical and surgical history; for example, a history of endometriosis, abdominal or testicular surgery which may affect the feasibility of the procedure. In addition, ask about any current conditions, such as anticoagulant use, which may require an alternative procedure or additional precautions during surgery.
- Current contraception – advice can be given regarding likely change in periods once this method is stopped.
- Menstrual history in women which may suggest a more appropriate method of contraception; for example, a history of heavy menstrual bleeding for which a levonorgestrel IUS would be an effective method of managing symptoms and providing long-term contraception.
- Failure rate.
- Discussion of the fact that there are other highly effective methods such as long-acting reversible contraception (LARC).
- Irreversibility.
- Time until the procedure is effective and the minimum length of time that current reliable contraception should be continued. There is no need to stop CHC prior to surgery.

- Details of the procedures, use of anaesthetic and the risks and benefits, complications and the myths associated with them. Provide written information to support the details given in the consultation; these can be accessed from www. rcog.org.uk or www.nhs.uk.
- Inform both partners that, compared to female sterilization by laparotomy or laparoscopy, vasectomy:
  - is more effective
  - is safer
  - is quicker to perform
  - is associated with less morbidity
  - requires only a local anaesthetic.
- When hysteroscopic sterilization is available:
  - discuss this option because there is reduced morbidity and no need for general anaesthesia compared to female sterilization by laparotomy or laparoscopy
  - indicate that it is irreversible
  - give pre-procedure advice such as analgesia and continuance of reliable contraception (excluding condoms due to their lower efficacy rate compared to other methods) until correct positioning of the implants is confirmed.
- These methods provide no protection against STIs.
- Male or female genital examination is advised to exclude potential problems such as a hydrocele, non-palpable vas deferens, gynaecological pathology, or evidence of previous surgery.

12.6 Regret

Evidence indicates that men and women are more likely to regret sterilization if they were under 30, have had no children, were not in a relationship or have relationship problems, or are sterilized immediately post-partum or post-abortion. In light of this, young and single people often receive additional counselling and may need to be reviewed by two specialists (rather than the typical one) who can obtain consent for the chosen procedure before it is undertaken.

Emotional problems including psychosexual dysfunction are more likely post-procedure if an individual is not absolutely certain about their decision at the time of the procedure.

12.7 Practical aspects

12.7.1 Vasectomy

This method of sterilization aims to prevent sperm entering the ejaculate through interruption of the vas deferens.

Efficacy

- Approximately 1 in 2000 male sterilizations fail after clearance has been confirmed by a post-vasectomy semen analysis; this equates to a failure rate of 0.05%.
- Compared to laparoscopic female sterilization, vasectomy is 30 times less likely to fail and 20 times less likely to be associated with post-operative complications.

Procedure

There are a variety of techniques for vasectomy, two of which are detailed below. Irrespective of the method chosen, the procedure typically takes 10–15 minutes to complete.

Conventional vasectomy:

- The scrotal skin is anaesthetized and two small incisions approximately 1 cm long are made.
- The incision provides access to the vas deferens which is cut and a small section removed. The ends of the vas deferens are ligated with sutures or cauterized.
- The incision is then closed, often with absorbable sutures such as Vicryl Rapide.

Minimally invasive vasectomy (MIV) (incorporating no-scalpel vasectomy (NSV) techniques):

- The vas deferens is located by palpation. Following infiltration with local anaesthetic, the vas deferens is then held in place by a small clamp.
- The skin of the scrotum is punctured on one side and forceps are used to open the incision site. A loop of vas deferens is then drawn through the incision. The vas deferens is interrupted and a section (1–3 cm long) is removed. Routine histological analysis of the removed section is not recommended.
- The upper and lower ends of the divided vas deferens are ligated or cauterized. Fascial interposition can be used as an adjunctive procedure.
- The second vas deferens can be accessed, divided and ligated or cauterized through the original puncture site.
- With this approach the opening in the scrotum is very small and may not require sutures to close.

The MIV techniques (as shown in *Figure 12.1*) are thought to be less painful and less likely to cause post-operative complications than a conventional vasectomy. Furthermore, cauterization is associated with a lower failure rate than ligation. The failure rate can be reduced by 50% with fascial interposition.

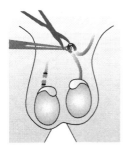

Figure 12.1. MIV vasectomy.

Post-procedure advice

- Men are advised to take a day or so off work if they have a sedentary job and up to a week off for those who have a manual job.
- Abstinence from sexual intercourse is recommended for 2–7 days.

- Firm scrotal support in the form of well-fitting underwear should be worn day and night for the first few days to reduce the risk of haematoma development.
- NSAIDs can be taken for post-operative pain unless there are personal contraindications.
- A semen analysis is ideally undertaken 12 weeks post-procedure (only one sample is required if the sample shows azoospermia).
- Advise patients to contact their healthcare provider if there is persistent bleeding, pain, possible infection or rapidly enlarging one-sided scrotal haematoma.

Risks and complications

- Mild testicular discomfort, swelling or bruising are common for the first few days following a vasectomy and can generally be managed by simple analgesics.
- Haematospermia (blood in semen) is common in the first few ejaculates after a vasectomy.
- Scrotal haematoma (minor bleeding 1:400, major bleeding 1:1000).
- Infection (1:100).
- Epididymitis (1:100).
- Sperm granuloma (1:500) – due to sperm leaking from the vas deferens into the surrounding tissues. It presents as a tender scrotal swelling near the proximal end of the vas deferens; excision may be required (1:500).
- Chronic pain (1:1000) can develop immediately following vasectomy or months to a year later. The pain is long-standing but not necessarily constant. It may occur occasionally or more frequently and can vary from a dull ache to a sharp pain. NSAIDs and treatment to alleviate neuropathic pain are common first-line treatment options. When this fails, further surgery involving reversal of vasectomy may be required, although pain may persist in a few cases.
- Failure to identify or locate one of the vas deferens – unilateral vasectomy can be undertaken followed by semen analysis at 12 weeks post-procedure. Referral for renal ultrasound to exclude ipsilateral renal agenesis is recommended.
- Where apparent bilateral absence of the vas deferens is encountered:
  - men should be referred for further investigation
  - if a double or duplicate vas deferens is found or suspected, arrange Doppler ultrasound to determine if it is a 'true' double vas deferens or an ectopic ureter. A renal and bladder ultrasound can also be arranged.
- There is currently no evidence of a causal relationship between vasectomy and prostate cancer and no increased risk of testicular cancer.
- Failure of the procedure has occurred if motile sperm are still seen 7 months post-surgery. In a small minority of men non-motile sperm are found in a specimen 7 months after vasectomy. Special clearance can be given to stop additional contraceptive methods when less than 100 000 non-motile sperm/ml are observed in a fresh semen sample.
- Late failure due to vas recanalization occurs in 0.03–1.2% of previously effective vasectomies.

Common misconceptions

- **Vasectomy causes cancer** – there is no evidence of a causal relationship between vasectomy and prostate or testicular cancer.

- **Vasectomy causes weight gain, hair loss or reduced strength** – vasectomy has no effect on male hormone levels; men look and feel the same as prior to the procedure.
- **Vasectomy results in a loss of sexual function and sex drive** - vasectomy does not affect the sexual drive, nor does it affect a man's ability to get an erection, have sex, or ejaculate. In fact, now that the risk of pregnancy has been removed sexual pleasure may actually increase.
- **Vasectomy alters the amount and appearance of the ejaculate** – this is not true because most of the ejaculate is made up of secretions from the seminal vesicles, prostate gland and Cowper's glands; this does not change post-vasectomy – only the sperm are absent.
- **Vasectomy reversal is always effective** – vasectomy reversal requires complex surgery and although high patency rates are achieved, a return to fertility may not occur. The longer the duration from vasectomy to reversal, the lower the patency and pregnancy rates.

12.7.2 Laparoscopic sterilization (tubal occlusion)

This method of sterilization involves preventing an ovum reaching the uterus by clipping, cutting and ligating, or applying rings to the Fallopian tubes.

It can be undertaken at any time providing the woman attending has abstained from sexual intercourse since her last menstrual period or is correctly using an effective method of contraception. If there is concern regarding a potential pregnancy the procedure should be delayed until the follicular phase of the next menstrual cycle.

Efficacy

- The lifetime failure rate for laparoscopic sterilization is 1 in 200.
- The 10 year failure rate for sterilization using Filshie clips appears to be lower at 1:333–500. However, patients should be aware that if the procedure fails there is an increased risk of ectopic pregnancy.

Procedure

Currently the recommended method of laparoscopic sterilization is with mechanical occlusion of the Fallopian tubes by applying Filshie clips to the Fallopian tubes. This method is less likely than alternatives to lead to complications.

- Pre-operatively a pregnancy test is undertaken along with recording of last menstrual period and current method of contraception.
- A standard laparoscopic approach is taken, with insufflation of the abdomen and then insertion of a port sub-umbilically. Once the laparoscope is passed through the port site the abdominal wall can be visualized and a second port can be introduced under direct vision in the suprapubic region.
- The Fallopian tubes are then identified and clips are applied across the narrowest portion of the tube, 1–2 cm from the cornu, to occlude the Fallopian tubes. Alternatives to clips include rings or occasionally bipolar diathermy if mechanical techniques fail.

Mini-laparotomy

A mini-laparotomy is an alternative approach.

- A small transverse incision just above the pubic symphysis (typically 4 cm above) is made.
- The Fallopian tubes are identified and a small portion removed (salpingectomy) or the tubes are occluded with clips or rings.
- There is less chance of reversal with tubal diathermy or salpingectomy than with other techniques.

A mini-laparotomy may be recommended for women who:

- Have had recent abdominal or pelvic surgery.
- Are obese.
- Have a history of pelvic inflammatory disease.
- Immediately post-partum or if the procedure is undertaken at the time of Caesarean section.
- As an alternative if a laparoscopic approach fails.

Post-procedure advice

- The majority of women return home on the day of the procedure.
- Women are advised to take 5–7 days off work depending on their occupation.
- If any intra-operative complications occur during the procedure both the patient and GP should be informed.
- If abdominal pain increases or an individual feels increasingly unwell they are advised to seek urgent medical help because these symptoms may suggest a perforation to bowel, bladder or blood vessels.

Potential complications

- Failure to gain entry into the abdomen, with 1 in 500 risk of a laparotomy being performed as a consequence of a severe complication during a laparoscopic procedure.
- Injury to bowel, bladder and or blood vessels (2–3 per 1000); this risk is increased in obese women, those with adhesions or endometriosis, or those who have previously undergone abdominal or pelvic surgery or have pelvic inflammatory disease.
- Risk of death with laparoscopy is 1 in 12 000 procedures.
- Uterine perforation (1:1000).
- Infection.
- Haemorrhage.
- Bruising.
- Abdominal and shoulder pain is common and normally caused by creating a pneumoperitoneum during surgery. This gradually settles during the week following the procedure.
- Moderate to severe abdominal pain is reported in up to 63% of women post-operatively, with 27% of women experiencing milder pain, and 50% experience mild pain at 3 months post-procedure.

- There is no evidence that sterilization results in heavier or more painful periods; however, women have often used hormonal methods of contraception prior to their sterilization which lightens menstrual loss and decreases dysmenorrhoea.
- Failure of procedure. If the procedure fails, any resulting pregnancy may be ectopic. (The incidence of ectopic pregnancy depends upon the method used to occlude the tubes. A recent study suggests a 10% ectopic rate if sterilization fails. Ectopic pregnancies are more common in women who have had diathermy to their Fallopian tubes rather than part of their tube removed or a clip placed over the tube.)
- If reversal of sterilization for pregnancy is requested, a Fallopian tube re-anastomosis can be undertaken as a private procedure; this procedure is associated with high tubal patency rates, but this may still not result in a pregnancy.

12.7.3 Hysteroscopic sterilization

Hysteroscopic sterilization is an outpatient transcervical sterilization procedure. In the UK the only licensed device approved by NICE is Essure.

Efficacy

Many studies examining the efficacy of hysteroscopic sterilization are methodologically flawed and limited by lack of longitudinal data, and so pregnancy rates vary; they are thought to be about 1 in 1000 over a 5 year period. The failure rate increases to 1 in 500 if one includes those who were in early luteal phase pregnancy or did not use additional reliable contraception until procedure success was confirmed.

Procedure

- Pre-operatively a pregnancy test is undertaken along with recording of last menstrual period and current method of contraception.
- There is no need to remove an IUC prior to the procedure. However, women should be advised to abstain from sexual intercourse for 7 days before surgery in case the IUC needs to be removed to access the tubal ostia.
- A hysteroscope is passed through the cervix and into the uterus. Ideally a vaginoscopic approach is undertaken, wherein the hysteroscope is introduced into the cervix without the use of a speculum, with the aim of reducing the pain associated with the procedure.
- The uterine cavity is inspected and the ostia identified.
- A flexible micro-insert on a guide wire is passed through a channel in the hysteroscope into each Fallopian tube.
- The micro-inserts induce a benign fibrotic reaction within the Fallopian tubes, which eventually blocks them (*Figure 12.2*).
- The procedure typically takes 10 minutes to perform.
- Additional contraception should be used until follow-up at approximately 3 months post-procedure. An IUC should not be introduced at the time of sterilization.

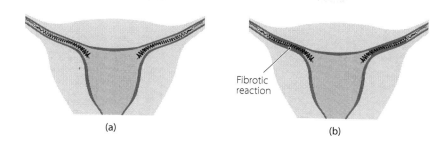

Figure 12.2. The use of the Essure micro-insert induces a fibrotic reaction within the Fallopian tubes. (a) Before fibrosis and (b) after fibrosis. © Bayer. Figure reproduced with the kind permission of Bayer.

Routine follow-up following hysteroscopic sterilization

- Three months post-procedure imaging, normally using ultrasound or X-ray (hysterosalpingogram is an alternative), is undertaken to confirm that the micro-inserts are correctly positioned.

Potential complications

1. Increased risk of ectopic pregnancy (up to 50%) if pregnancy occurs.
2. Intra- and post-operative pain. Acute severe post-operative pelvic pain occurs in 8.1% of women, with milder pain reported in 79% of women.
3. Infection.
4. Bleeding – approximately one-third of women bleed and two-thirds have spotting for up to 3 days post-procedure.
5. Perforation of the uterus (1:1000) or of the Fallopian tube with the micro-insert (1–3 per 100).
6. Failure to place one or both of the micro-inserts (1–14% cases).
7. Incorrect insertion of the implant (2:100).
8. Chronic pelvic pain – there may an increased risk of developing post-procedure pain in women with pre-existing pain. The incidence of chronic pelvic pain is 0.16%.
9. There is no evidence of an increased risk of ovarian cancer and limited evidence suggests the procedure may have a protective effect.
10. There is no evidence of an association with sterilization and endometrial, cervical or breast cancer.
11. It is not possible to reverse micro-insert sterilization via Fallopian tube anastamosis and so *in vitro* fertilization (IVF) would be advised if pregnancy is sought. Studies of success rates for IVF following hysteroscopic sterilization are limited but case series suggest an overall pregnancy rate of 27% per cycle; however, these studies were underpowered and subject to bias.

12.8 Myths and misconceptions

- **Female sterilization causes cancer** – sterilization does not increase the risk of cancer; indeed, several studies have reported a reduced risk of ovarian cancer after tubal occlusion. Very little research has been done to investigate the relationship between breast cancer and female sterilization, but so far there is no evidence of such a link.
- **Female sterilization stops ovulation and affects hormones** – sterilization acts to block the Fallopian tubes to prevent the ovum entering the uterus. It does not prevent ovulation. In addition, female hormones are not affected and so there is neither a loss of femininity nor any change in sexual functioning.
- **Female sterilization causes periods to become more painful, heavier or more irregular** – as sterilization has no effect on hormonal function there is no effect on an individual's menstrual cycle. Women often use hormonal contraceptives prior to sterilization which generally lightens periods and helps period pain; combined hormonal methods also regulate the cycle.
- **Female sterilization causes weight gain and loss of sex drive** – there is no evidence that sterilization affects weight, appetite or physical appearance; however, weight gain is more common in older women and this group is more likely to undergo sterilization. Neither procedure has an effect on sexual desire or function – in fact women may find sexual pleasure increases once they do not have to worry about pregnancy risk.

EXAMPLE

A 39 year old woman who has 2 children attends requesting sterilization because she is looking for a long-term method of contraception. She has a past medical history of endometriosis which has been investigated with a laparoscopy.

What questions you would ask and what are the management options?

1. Ideally you would see the woman with her partner.
2. You would take a complete medical and surgical history, along with current contraception and current gynaecological symptoms. Determine if the children are with current partner and ensure her family is complete.
3. Identify reasons for requesting the sterilization.
4. Discuss alternatives to sterilization such as LARC.
5. Discuss advantages and disadvantages and potential complications of the methods.
6. If sterilization is chosen as the method of contraception, vasectomy or hysteroscopic sterilization would be the safer options in this case.

References

FSRH (2014) *Male and Female Sterilisation*. Clinical Effectiveness Unit [www.fsrh.org/documents/cec-ceu-guidance-sterilisation-summary-sep-2014/ – accessed June 2016]

Health and Social Care Information Centre (HSCIC) (2012) *NHS Contraceptive Services: England, 2011/12*. Community Contraceptive Clinics. Leeds, UK.

Information Services Division (2011) *Sterilisation Key Clinical Indicator (KCI)*. Year ending December 2010. Edinburgh, UK.

Mijatovic, V. *et al.* (2012) Essure hydrosalpinx occlusion prior to IVF-ET as an alternative to laparoscopic salpingectomy. *Eur. J. Obstet. Gynecol. Reprod. Biol.* **161**: 42–45.

Chapter 13
Emergency contraception

Emergency contraception (EC) is taken after sex has occurred, to prevent an unintended pregnancy. It is also known as post-coital contraception or the 'morning after pill'. EC is used by 7% of women each year in the UK. Because no method of contraception is perfect, EC is an important back-up for all. Accessing EC is often felt to be difficult due to the stigma women perceive to be associated with its use.

There are three forms of EC currently available in the UK:
- oral progestogen-only EC – levonorgestrel
- oral selective progesterone receptor modulator – ulipristal acetate (UPA)
- copper IUD.

EC may be needed because contraception was not used, or because of a contraception failure such as forgotten progestogen-only or combined contraceptive pills, expulsion of an intrauterine contraceptive, or failure of a barrier method (see *Table 13.2* later in this chapter for possible indications for EC). EC is not an abortifacient and, with the exception of the copper IUD, does not provide ongoing contraception.

Previously, an oral combined oestrogen and progestogen preparation containing 100 mcg ethinyl oestradiol and 1 mg levonorgestrel taken 12 hours apart (the Yupze method) was used; however, this is less effective than progestogen-only EC and is no longer available in the UK. Mifepristone may be used as an EC; however, it is not licensed in the UK.

13.1 Potential users

13.1.1 Most appropriate users

- All women with no contraindications should be offered an IUD because it is the most effective method of EC.
- There are no medical contraindications to the levonorgestrel EC.

13.1.2 Not suitable for the following users

The copper IUD is not suitable for those:
- more than 2 days but less than 4 weeks post-partum
- with persistently elevated β-hCG levels following gestational trophoblastic or malignant disease
- with uterine cavity distortion – an attempt may be undertaken after careful counselling
- with current pelvic inflammatory disease
- with a history of copper allergy.

Oral methods of EC are affected by liver enzyme inducing drugs (see *Table 3.1*), and so an IUD is the method of choice for those using these medications. However, if an IUD is contraindicated, double dose (3 mg) of levonorgestrel can be prescribed (off licence but supported by national guidance from the Faculty of Sexual and Reproductive Healthcare (FSRH, 2012)).

UPA is not recommended for women who are:
- hypersensitive to UPA
- pregnant
- severe asthmatics which is insufficiently controlled by oral steroids
- suffering from hepatic dysfunction
- galactose intolerant, lactase deficient or have glucose–galactose malabsorption
- breast-feeding (not recommended for 7 days after UPA use – milk should be expressed and discarded)
- using medications which increase gastric pH such as antacids, histamine antagonists and proton pump inhibitors because absorption and efficacy are reduced.

13.2 Available emergency contraception in the UK

Doses and indications for a range of EC products are provided in *Table 13.1*.

13.3 Mechanism of action

13.3.1 Copper IUD

- The main mode of action when used as EC is inhibition of fertilization. If fertilization has already occurred, the IUD has an anti-implantation effect.
- It is effective immediately as an ongoing method of contraception.

13.3.2 Levonorgestrel

- The mechanism of action is not completely understood but is thought to be primarily by inhibition of ovulation. Ovulation is delayed for 5–7 days by which time any sperm in the reproductive tract will be non-viable.
- When taken prior to the luteinizing hormone (LH) surge, ovulation is delayed or inhibited. The closer to ovulation treatment is given, the lower the probability of this method preventing pregnancy (see *Figure 13.1*).

Table 13.1. EC available in the UK

Method	Products	Recommended dose	Licensed indication
Copper-bearing IUD (containing at least 300 mm² of copper)	Various types are licensed for contraception but not for EC (approximately £10)	Retained until pregnancy excluded, e.g. onset of period or at least 3 weeks after unprotected sex, or for the licensed duration of the IUD	Within 5 days (120 hours) of first episode of unprotected sex or within 5 days of the earliest estimated date of ovulation
Levonorgestrel (progestogen)	*Levonelle One Step* £13.83 POM £22–28 P *Levonelle 1500* £5.20 POM £25.99–£27 P *Upostelle* £3.75 POM £13.83 P	1.5 mg single oral dose	Within 72 hours of unprotected sex or contraception failure or, off licence, up to 96 hours after unprotected sex
Ulipristal acetate (UPA) (progestogen receptor modulator)	*ellaOne* £13.83 POM £34.95 P	30 mg single oral dose	Within 120 hours of unprotected sex or contraception failure

Data from *British National Formulary* 2015, or direct from manufacturers (2015)
P = pharmacy medicine (available without prescription; prices may vary depending on location),
POM = prescription only medicine.

- If fertilization has occurred, levonorgestrel has no effect on pregnancy prevention. It is not known to adversely affect pregnancy outcome.
- Levonorgestrel is licensed for use up to 72 hours after unprotected sex, but it may be taken up to 96 hours after unprotected sex (off licence).
- Resume or start contraception with additional barrier method cover as specified in *Table 13.3*.

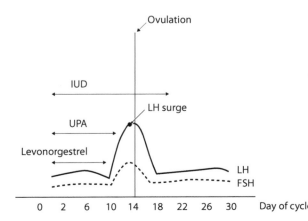

Figure 13.1. Efficacy of EC in relation to ovulation. The lines on the graph indicate the times during which a method is most likely to be effective. If the LH surge has not yet started all three methods may be effective in preventing pregnancy. Once the LH surge has started only UPA and the IUD are beneficial. Following the LH peak an IUD is the most efficacious.

13.3.3 Ulipristal acetate (UPA)

- UPA is a selective progesterone receptor modulator with antagonistic and partial agonistic effects. It binds to progesterone receptors in target tissues: the uterus, ovaries and hypothalamus.
- Its main mode of action is inhibition or delay of ovulation. If the LH surge has started but not peaked, ovulation can be prevented, with up to a 5 day delay in follicular rupture.
- Administration at the time of or after the LH surge has no effect in delaying follicular rupture.
- Women should wait 5 whole days after using UPA before starting or recommencing hormonal contraception, as current evidence suggests concurrent use may reduce the efficacy of the UPA. During this time and until effective contraceptive cover for their chosen method of contraception has been achieved (see *Table 13.3*) individuals should either abstain or use barrier methods.

13.4 Efficacy of emergency contraception

Studies suggest that the failure rate with the different types of EC varies as follows:
- with levonorgestrel the failure rate is between 1.7 and 2.2% if unprotected sex has occurred within the previous 72 hours
- with UPA the failure rate is between 1.3 and 1.6% if unprotected sex has occurred within the previous 120 hours; there is no decline in efficacy over the 120 hours following unprotected sex
- with an IUD used as EC very few women become pregnant ; one large study of nearly 2000 women reported no pregnancies in the first month after EC IUD fitting.

Ideally, therefore, an IUD should be offered first-line to all women who have no contraindications.

13.5 Provision of emergency contraception

When assessing the need for EC it is important to consider:
- LMP date
- usual cycle length and estimated date of ovulation (see *Figure 13.2*)

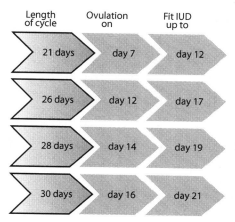

Length of cycle	Ovulation on	Fit IUD up to
21 days	day 7	day 12
26 days	day 12	day 17
28 days	day 14	day 19
30 days	day 16	day 21

Figure 13.2. How to calculate the period of time when an EC IUD can be fitted.

- the timing of **all** episodes of unprotected sex in the current cycle – the probability of pregnancy following sex during the first 3 days of the menstrual cycle appears to be negligible
- details of potential contraceptive failures, for example, how many missed pills and when in the packet (see *Table 13.2*)
- previous EC use in the cycle
- past medical history to determine medical eligibility
- medications used, including herbal medicines which may affect efficacy of oral EC
- the need for ongoing contraception, which should be discussed with all women attending for EC
- sexual history to determine risk of STIs (see *Chapter 14*).

Table 13.2. Indications for emergency contraception

Method of contraception	Possible contraceptive failure	Indications for EC
Combined hormonal or progestogen-only pill or implant	Failure to use additional contraceptive precautions whilst using liver enzyme inducing medication or in the 28 days following their use	If unprotected sex has occurred or barrier method fails Use IUD or double dose levonorgestrel (3mg)
Combined oral contraceptive	Two or more missed pills	EC is indicated if the pills were missed in week one of a packet and unprotected sex occurred during that 1st week or during the hormone-free week EC is indicated if the hormone-free interval is extended; an IUD can be fitted up to 15 days after the last active pill (providing all other pills had been taken correctly)
Combined contraceptive ring or patch	Extension of patch or ring-free interval by more than 48 hours	EC is indicated if sex occurred in the patch- or ring-free interval
	If patch or ring is detached or removed for more than 48 hours	EC should be considered if the patch or ring was detached or removed in week 1 and unprotected sex occurred in the patch- or ring-free week
Progestogen-only pill	Late or missed pills, i.e. more than 27 hours since last traditional pill or more than 36 hours since last desogestrel-containing pill	If there has been unprotected sex or a barrier failure since the missed pill and before efficacy is re-established, i.e. in the 48 hours after restarting the pill An IUD can be fitted up to 5 days after the unprotected sex or oral EC can be offered
Progestogen-only injectable	Late injection more than 14 weeks since last injection of DMPA	If all unprotected sex occurred in the last 5 days, an IUD may be fitted or oral EC used
Intrauterine methods	Removal without immediate replacement, partial or complete expulsion	If sex occurred in the 5 days before removal or expulsion it may be appropriate to fit an IUD or offer oral EC

All EC methods which are appropriate for the clinical circumstances should be offered and discussed, including their effectiveness, to enable the woman to select her preferred method.

- An IUD is the most effective option and therefore is generally first-line for all attending for EC.
- Take a pragmatic approach to providing oral EC. UPA may be particularly suitable for those who have had unprotected sex 72–120 hours before attendance and those within 3 days either side of the estimated date of ovulation.
- If an individual presents requiring EC between 72 and 120 hours after sex, but UPA is contraindicated and an IUD is declined, levonorgestrel may be used but its efficacy will be reduced. There is evidence suggesting that levonorgestrel EC has no effect after 96 hours.
- If EC is required more than once in a cycle and all episodes are within 5 days of an estimated date of ovulation, an IUD can be used. If an oral method is requested, levonorgestrel and UPA can be used more than once in a cycle (UKMEC 1).
- There is currently insufficient evidence to advocate the use of UPA in all obese women seeking oral EC, although concerns have been raised regarding reduced efficacy; obesity is a UKMEC 1 for all methods.

If a woman selects an IUD as her method of EC but it is not immediately available, oral EC should be given as an interim measure in case the IUD cannot be fitted or the woman fails to attend the appointment.

13.6 Provision of ongoing contraception

- Women may prefer to wait until pregnancy can be excluded before starting a hormonal method.
- Quick-starting an ongoing method of contraception (see *Chapter 1*) after EC can be considered for all women based on their medical eligibility and preference. *Tables 13.3* and *13.4* illustrate duration of additional contraception following use of levonorgestrel EC and UPA EC, respectively. Note that with UPA use, the chosen method of contraception should not be commenced until 5 whole days after EC.
- It is recommended that the progestogen-only injectable is quick-started only if all other methods are declined.
- The IUS should not be quick-started but a bridging method used until pregnancy can be excluded.

13.7 Routine follow-up

- Pregnancy test 3 weeks after the episode(s) of unprotected sex.
- Consider repeating offer of STI screening.
- Review IUD at 3 weeks if ongoing use is planned:
  - if the IUD is not required as long-term contraception it can be removed at the next period
  - if an alternative method of contraception is started on the first day of the next period then the IUD can be removed
  - if an alternative method is started at any other time the IUD could remain in place from 2 to 9 days (depending on the chosen contraceptive) until that method is effective.

Table 13.3. Duration of additional contraceptive required following use of levonorgestrel EC

Method of contraception started or recommenced	Duration of additional contraception following use of levonorgestrel EC
CHC including patch and vaginal ring	7 days
COC containing oestradiol valerate and dienogest	9 days
Progestogen-only implant	7 days
Progestogen-only injectable	7 days
Progestogen-only pill	2 days

Table 13.4. Duration of additional contraceptive required following use of UPA EC

Method of contraception started or recommenced	Delay required after UPA use before contraception can be started or recommenced	Duration of additional contraception following use of UPA EC
CHC including patch and vaginal ring	UPA given on Day 0 Advise women not to commence contraception until Day 6 after UPA use	7 days
COC containing oestradiol valerate and dienogest		9 days
Progestogen-only implant		7 days
Progestogen-only injectable		7 days
Progestogen-only pill		2 days

EXAMPLE

A 30 year old woman attends to discuss contraception because she wishes to start 'the pill'. Her LMP was 12 days earlier; it was a normal period. She typically has a 28 day cycle, has no medical conditions or contraindications and is not currently using any medication. She had a condom failure 2 days ago (day 10).

What should you discuss?

1. Check if any other episodes of unprotected sex have occurred during this cycle.
2. Any use of EC earlier in this cycle?
3. Sexual history to determine risk and offer STI testing as appropriate.
4. Discuss all EC options available: IUD, levonorgestrel and UPA.
5. Carefully discuss the efficacy of each method, explaining that the IUD is the most effective method of EC.
6. If she opts for an oral method, levonorgestrel would be an acceptable option.
7. If she wishes to quick-start an oral method of contraception following levonorgestrel EC, a POP could be commenced with additional contraception for 2 days or, if a CHC is preferred, 7 days of additional contraception would be required.
8. Follow-up for pregnancy test in 3 weeks.

13.8 Managing side-effects

- Nausea occurs in fewer than 20% of women following oral EC and vomiting in less than 1%. If vomiting occurs within 3 hours of taking UPA or levonorgestrel a further dose of EC is needed or an IUD could be fitted.
- The time of menses may be affected by EC. Most women bleed within 7 days of their expected period date. Menstruation occurs on average 1.2 days earlier than expected for users of levonorgestrel and on average 2 days later than expected when using UPA. Women should be advised that about 1 in 5 women have a period that is delayed for 7 days or more with UPA.
- Pain associated with insertion of an IUD may occur and this can generally be alleviated with simple analgesia and advice to return if pain fails to resolve or becomes severe.
- Other side-effects associated with oral EC include headache, dizziness, diarrhoea and breast tenderness, which all resolve quickly after use.

13.9 Myths and misconceptions

- **There is only one type of emergency contraception and it can only be used the morning after unprotected sex** – there are three methods of EC currently available in the UK and, potentially, they may all be suitable depending on the timing of unprotected sex. UPA and the IUD can be offered up to 5 days after unprotected sex.

EXAMPLE

A 19 year old woman attends requesting emergency contraception. She had unprotected sex the night before. Discussion reveals her LMP was 17 days earlier and she has a 28 day cycle. She also had unprotected sex on days 14, 12 and 10.

What should you do?

1. Determine medical history to assess medical eligibility.
2. Sexual history to determine risk and offer STI testing as appropriate.
3. As all sex occurred within 5 days of estimated date of ovulation (estimated date of ovulation is day 14 in in a 28 day cycle therefore an IUD could be fitted up to day 19), an IUD would be the most appropriate method of EC and may also be used for ongoing contraception.
4. Organize IUD fit if acceptable. Provide UPA if there are no contraindications and an IUD fitting cannot be undertaken immediately.
5. In an asymptomatic woman insertion of an IUD can be carried out without the need for prophylactic antibiotics, providing she is easily contactable and will re-attend if an infection is identified.
6. Prophylactic antibiotics for chlamydia (and gonorrhoea depending on local prevalence) can be considered in those at high risk of an STI.
7. Follow-up in approximately 3 weeks after next menses.

- **Emergency contraception causes an abortion** – this is not correct; EC works by delaying ovulation or preventing fertilization or implantation and so its action occurs before implantation occurs.
- **Emergency contraception causes infertility** – EC has a very short-term effect and there is no effect on future fertility.
- **Emergency contraception can only be used a small number of times in a woman's life** – there is not a maximum number of times EC can be used. EC can be used whenever it is needed. Frequent use of oral EC is not recommended, however, because it is not as effective as regular contraception but repeated use poses no health risks and has no effect on future fertility.
- **Emergency contraception should not be provided as an advanced supply** – this is not the case; research suggests that women who have EC in advance are more likely to use it and use it sooner after the episode of sex than those without an advanced supply. The provision of an advanced supply can be decided on a case-by-case basis for women who may be at risk; for example, those women using barrier methods or the withdrawal method.
- **If pregnancy occurs after emergency contraception use it needs to be managed differently to any other pregnancy** – for those who had an IUD inserted, the site of pregnancy should be determined by ultrasound scan and removal of the IUD before 12 weeks of pregnancy is recommended. An IUD left *in situ* during pregnancy is associated with miscarriage, preterm delivery, septic abortion and chorioamnionitis. Removal of the IUD improves the outcome. For those who used UPA, the pregnancy is reported to the manufacturers to enable monitoring of outcomes of exposure during pregnancy. Levonorgestrel is not known to have a harmful effect on pregnancy.

References

British National Formulary, September 2014–March 2015.

FSRH (2012) Emergency Contraception. Clinical Effectiveness Unit [www.fsrh.org/documents/ceu-emergency-contraception-jan-2012/ – accessed June 2016]

FSRH (2015) Statement from the Clinical Effectiveness Unit – Quick starting after UPA [www.fsrh.org/documents/ceustatementquickstartingafterupa/ – accessed June 2016]

UKMEC (2016) *UK Medical Eligibility Criteria for Contraceptive Use* [www.fsrh.org/standards-and-guidance/uk-medical-eligibility-criteria-for-contraceptive-use/ – accessed June 2016]

Chapter 14
STIs, safe sex and sexual assault

- Sexually transmitted infections (STIs) are infections passed from one person to another during sex or close sexual contact.
- The recognition of, and screening for, STIs are important components of sexual and reproductive health, irrespective of the setting in which a consultation takes place.
- There are no contraindications to the offer of testing for infections. In fact, if we offer testing as part of 'contraception' consultations, we increase the scope and acceptability of testing.

14.1 Potential users

Table 14.1 outlines the situations in which clinicians may wish to consider undertaking STI testing.

14.2 Sexual history taking

A sexual history is important in the assessment of risk and in determining which infections to test for and from which sites. Sexual health issues may present as a hidden agenda in a consultation. Individuals may be reluctant to discuss their health concerns due to fears of stigma.

Components of a sexual history include:
- Symptoms review – change in vaginal discharge, dysuria, skin changes, abdominal or pelvic pain, intermenstrual or post-coital bleeding.
- Previous sexual partners – all partners in the last 3–6 months, time of last episode of sex, gender of partner(s), condom use, type of sex (anal, oral or vaginal).
- Previous STIs – diagnosis, treatment, compliance with treatment and treatment of partner. Is there a risk of re-infection or failure of treatment?
- Last menstrual period, cycle length, intermenstrual bleeding, post-coital bleeding, contraceptive use and cervical sample history.

Table 14.1. When and to whom to offer STI testing

Situation	Description
On request from patient	• As part of sexual health many individuals now attend for a regular check-up based on their own perceived risk
Known at-risk individuals	• Under 25 years of age • New partner within the last 12 months • More than one partner in the previous 12 months • Intravenous drug user • From high-risk area for HIV or syphilis (e.g. sub-Saharan Africa, Russia and parts of South East Asia and the Caribbean) • Those who have paid for sex or who have been paid for sex • Those who have had a blood transfusion in the UK pre-1992 or surgery/transfusion abroad • Those who have high-risk partner, i.e. partner who has an STI, who has multiple sexual partners, who is bisexual, who uses intravenous drugs, or from high HIV or syphilis-prevalent country • Those who have a clinical indicator disease for HIV as outlined in the UK national guidelines for HIV testing, such as cervical intra-epithelia neoplasia grade 2 or above, oral candidiasis, pyrexia of unknown origin (see www.bhiva.org/HIV-testing-guidelines.aspx for further details)
Symptomatic patients	• With increase or change in vaginal discharge • With dysuria • With intermenstrual or post-coital bleeding • With pelvic or abdominal pain • With dyspareunia
Pre-procedure	• Before abortion • Before insertion of intrauterine contraception, endometrial sample, hysteroscopy in known at-risk groups
Screening programme	• Chlamydia screening programme for all sexually active women and men under the age of 25 years

• Blood-borne virus risk assessment, including history of blood transfusion (pre-1992), surgery, injection or blood transfusions outside the UK, intravenous drug use by self or partner, any other recreational drug usage, partner(s) from overseas, partner(s) who have sex with men, being paid or paying for sex, known blood-borne virus infection in partner.
• Means of providing the results of investigations, e.g. text, letter.
• Assess for vulnerability, risk of exploitation or child protection concerns.

There are a variety of testing kits and several laboratory platforms available for infection testing.
• They differ with regard to transportation and refrigeration and so a discussion with local laboratory services is recommended.
• The gold standard tests and, where applicable, alternative tests for the most common infections are outlined in *Table 14.2* along with incubation periods and/or window periods, first-line treatment and recommended follow-up.
• Testing should not be delayed until the end of a window period. Instead individuals should be tested at time of presentation and advised of the need for repeat testing if last sexual partner was within the window period.

Table 14.2. Testing, window/incubation periods, treatment and follow-up for common STIs

Infection	Test	Window or incubation period since last UPSI	Treatment	Repeat testing
Chlamydia trachomatis	NAAT* – self-taken vulvo-vaginal swab in women and urine sample in men (1–2 hours since last passed urine, depending on testing kit); laboratories undertake confirmatory testing on all positive results to reduce the false positive rate	2 weeks	Azithromycin 1 g orally as a single dose OR Doxycycline 100 mg orally twice daily for 7 days If pregnant or breast-feeding: • erythromycin 500 mg four times a day for 7 days OR • erythromycin 500 mg twice a day for 14 days OR • amoxicillin 500 mg three times a day for 7 days OR • azithromycin 1 g as a single dose orally	Not routinely needed unless: • the woman receiving treatment is pregnant (due to reduced efficacy of treatment) • compliance issues are suspected NAAT testing is repeated 6 weeks after azithromycin or 5 weeks after doxycycline treatment • In under 25s repeat testing is recommended 3 months after treatment in case they have a newly acquired infection
Neisseria gonorrhoeae	NAAT – following positive diagnosis a culture specimen should be taken to enable identification of antibiotic sensitivity	3–14 days (convention is to undertake testing at the same time as chlamydia testing)	Ceftriaxone 500 mg single dose IM injection plus azithromycin 1 g single dose orally OR Spectinomycin 2 g single dose IM injection for penicillin-allergic individuals	A repeat NAAT swab is recommended 2 weeks after treatment if diagnosis is made by NAAT as a 'test of cure'

Infection	Test	Window or incubation period since last UPSI	Treatment	Repeat testing
Trichomonas vaginalis	NAAT (or culture broth if NAAT not available); may be identified as part of cervical screening (smears)	Unknown; however, *in vitro* studies suggest 4–28 days	Metronidazole 400 mg orally twice a day for 7 days OR Metronidazole 2 g orally as a single dose (avoid single high dose in breast-feeding)	Not required unless the individual remains symptomatic after treatment
HIV	Clotted blood for both HIV antibodies and p24 antigen (a 4th generation HIV test): p24 antigen is a protein which makes up most of the viral core; concentrations of p24 are high in the first few weeks of infection; antibodies to p24 are produced following seroconversion and so p24 is generally undetectable after seroconversion after initial infection antibodies to HIV antigens begin to appear in the blood; screening test looks for antibodies to HIV surface proteins	4 weeks (8 weeks in high risk exposure; 8–12 weeks following an assault, the later if PEPSE has been taken)	Anti-retroviral therapy depending on CD4 count and patient request	Monitoring and follow-up will depend on response to treatment and general health
Syphilis	Clotted blood for serological testing to look for treponemal antibodies (including syphilis); a screening test or full syphilis serology may be requested: all individuals with	Incubation period 9–90 days; end of window period is 12 weeks after exposure	For early syphilis (primary, secondary or early latent) benzathine penicillin G 2.4 million units IM as a single dose OR doxycycline 100 mg orally twice daily for 14 days	For early syphilis, clinical and serological follow-up at 1, 2, 3, 6 and 12 months, then 6 monthly until Rapid Plasma Reagin (RPR) test or the

Infection	Test	Window or incubation period since last UPSI	Treatment	Repeat testing
Syphilis (*cont.*)	previous infection with syphilis should always have a full syphilis screen (not always available in general practice) syphilis PCR testing on a swab taken from a chancre if identified on examination		For late syphilis: • benzathine penicillin 2.4 million units IM weekly for 2 weeks • (three doses) OR • doxycycline 100 mg orally twice daily for 28 days	Venereal Disease Research Laboratory (VDRL) test are negative or serofast (levels or VDRL or RPR remain static); these are non-specific quantitative tests which correlate with disease activity For late syphilis serological follow-up is 3 monthly until serofast
Genital warts (human papillomavirus)	Visual inspection or biopsy if any doubt about diagnosis	Variable from 3 months to several years	No treatment or • Cryotherapy • Podophyllotoxin 0.15% cream – topically twice a day for 3 days, followed by 4 days with no treatment for 4–5 cycles. • Imiquimod 5% – 3 times weekly for up to 16 weeks	Review at end of treatment or if change of treatment is required or if relapse occurs
Genital herpes (herpes simplex virus)	Visual inspection, NAAT for confirmation and typing (use of serology for antibodies to herpes simplex virus is limited)	2–14 days, however, testing is only undertaken if symptomatic	• Saline baths • Analgesia • Topical anaesthetic (5% lidocaine ointment) • Aciclovir 400 mg orally 3 times a day for 5 days OR valaciclovir 500 mg orally twice daily (only indicated if presentation is within 5 days of start of episode)	Not indicated

*NAAT – nucleic acid amplification test

14.3 Partner notification

- An important public health component of STI testing is partner notification. Its aim is to reduce or stop the onward transmission of infection through the identification, testing and, if appropriate, treatment of others known to be at risk as a result of sexual contact with the index case (i.e. the individual who was initially diagnosed).
- The process of partner notification involves identifying contacts who may have been at risk of infection and agreeing who will inform the contacts, the index case or a healthcare provider, for example, in primary care or via a GUM clinic anonymously. Finally, follow-up of the outcomes of partner notification is recommended.
- Partner notification begins at the time of diagnosis and treatment. The clinic or practice undertaking the initial testing and/or treatment does not necessarily need to complete the partner notification. However, discussion of the process involved and the importance of partner notification is recommended. A referral can be made to a local sexual health service which can facilitate the process of partner notification; alternatively, a partner notification contact slip(s) (see *Figure 14.1* for an example of a contact slip) may be given to the index patient for them to distribute to their contacts.
- Face-to-face or telephone consultations can be undertaken to provide support and advice to contacts about the possibility of infection and the provision of treatment if appropriate.

14.4 Sexual health advice

Safe sex is the means of taking responsibility for oneself by taking steps to reduce the risk of STIs and unplanned pregnancy. Sexual history taking can help identify those undertaking risky sexual behaviour who may benefit from a brief behaviour change intervention. Brief interventions have been shown to reduce STI incidence and increase condom usage.

Safe sex advice includes verbal and written information on:
- Condom efficacy and limitations (see *Chapter 10*).
- Condom types and sizes – ensure the condom is the correct size, particularly with regard to penis circumference, and is not too tight.
- Determinants of condom effectiveness.
- Use condoms for all episodes of sex including oral sex with advice that, while oral sex is lower risk than vaginal or anal sex, it is not risk free. If condoms are not used for every episode of sex, some use is safer than no use.
- STI testing is recommended before having sex with someone new and advising new partners to undergo testing even if they have no symptoms.
- Reducing the number of partners to reduce infection risk. This risk reduction, in terms of prevalence of infection, may be greater than that associated with increased condom use.
- Risk of transmission in penetrative sex including fingering, using sex toys and fisting relates to the degree of trauma experienced by an individual.

Contact slip

Instructions – please give this slip to your sexual partner(s) and advise them to take it to their GP or sexual health clinic. Do not have sex with your partner(s) until they have received treatment.

Dear ....

This letter is to inform you that you have been in contact with someone who has

....

This is a treatable sexually transmitted infection. Often people with this infection feel well and have no symptoms.

It is very important that you are tested and treated. Therefore please take this letter to either of the following places:

- Your general practice
- Sexual health clinic at ....

••

Please inform us that the contact attended your service

GP practice / Sexual health clinic details

Figure 14.1. Example of a partner notification contact slip.

- Avoid brushing teeth or flossing before oral sex.
- Avoid oral sex if cuts, sores or cold sores (oral herpes) are present on the mouth of the individual giving oral sex or if that individual has a sore throat. While oral sex is lower risk than vaginal or anal sex it is not risk-free.
- In addition, a condom demonstration and discussion regarding condom problems can be beneficial. Issues to discuss include:
  - removing air from tip of the condom
  - pulling back foreskin before putting on the condom to reduce the risk of condom slipping off or tearing
  - the fact that use of additional lubricant may double the risk of condom slippage
  - thicker condoms are no less likely to break or slip during anal sex than standard condoms.

14.5 Sexual assault

A compassionate and pragmatic approach is required when an individual presents following a sexual assault. An individual may attend immediately after the assault or after some considerable time, or at any point in between. The needs of the individual may be affected by the duration of time since the event.

14.5.1 Documentation, evidence and assessment

- A brief history of the event is documented verbatim including what time, when, where and by whom.
- If the assault was within the last 7 days management of any injuries sustained may be required. In addition, consideration and discussion of forensic medical examination to gather evidence is recommended. Forensic examinations are undertaken in Sexual Assault Referral Centres (SARC): swabs for DNA can be taken (see Table 14.3 for DNA evidence collection timing), injuries documented, and immediate medical care such as emergency contraception, HIV prophylaxis and hepatitis B vaccination can be provided. SARCs vary across the country and so it is advisable to check on the services offered locally. Generally an individual can self-refer and the police do not always need to be involved; evidence can be stored for later use.

Table 14.3. DNA forensic sample timetable

Site	Time up to which DNA can be detected
Vaginal	7 days after
Anal	3 days after
Oral	2 days after
Digital penetration	12 hours after

- If an individual presents immediately after the event they are advised not to shower or bathe, brush their teeth or wash their clothes. All clothes should be kept along with any pads or tampons worn at the time of the assault as they may provide evidence.
- An assessment of psychological wellbeing with particular reference to risk of self-harm and suicide is advisable. In addition, it is important to ascertain if it is safe to allow the individual to go home or if emergency accommodation is required and if there are any ongoing child or vulnerable adult protection issues.
- Some services undertake baseline STI screens while others wait until 2 weeks after the assault for chlamydia and gonorrhoea, and 3 months for HIV, syphilis and hepatitis B and C.
- Prophylactic antibiotics can be provided to women with a history of sexual assault; this reduces the need for testing and the chance of missing an infection if the individual defaults from follow-up. However, this approach may result in unnecessary treatment and reduces the potential for partner notification and increases the chance of re-infection if the original infection was from someone other than the assailant.

14.5.2 Hepatitis vaccination

Although the acquisition of hepatitis from sexual assault in the UK is uncommon, vaccination may be given up to 6 weeks after the assault in the following circumstances:
- Assailant known to be hepatitis B carrier.
- Assailant has risk factor(s), for example, intravenous drug users or man who has sex with men.
- Anal assault.
- Trauma and bleeding following the assault.
- Multiple assailants.
- Client wishes to have vaccination.

The vaccination may be given on day 0, 7 and 21 or day 0, at 1 month and at 2 months following the assault. Either regimen is followed by a booster at 1 year.

14.5.3 HIV infection and treatment

For individuals presenting within 72 hours of the assault, post-exposure prophylaxis after sexual exposure (PEPSE) to HIV can be considered based on an assessment of the risk of transmission, which is determined from the assailant's likelihood of having HIV and the risk of exposure (see *Figure 14.2* and *Table 14.5*). It is recommended that an individual is advised that there is a lack of conclusive data regarding the efficacy of PEPSE. Its side-effects, the length of treatment (28 days), the importance of adhering to treatment, and the frequency of follow-up should also be discussed. PEPSE can often be obtained from A&E departments or from sexual health services if not available at a SARC, or if the individual does not wish to attend a SARC. Prior to commencing PEPSE, a baseline HIV test is recommended.
- The currently recommended regimen for PEPSE is raltegravir/Truvada for 28 days. One Truvada tablet (245 mg tenofovir disoproxil (as fumarate) and 200 mg emtricitabine (FTC)) once a day plus one raltegravir tablet (400 mg) twice a day.
- If PEPSE is provided, HIV testing is recommended 3 months after the completion of treatment (4 months after the assault). (See *Table 14.4*)

Table 14.4. Recommended monitoring during PEPSE course and follow-up

	Baseline	14 days	8–12 weeks post-exposure
HIV	✔		✔
Hep B sAg (if no history of vaccination)	✔		✔ Only if not immune
STI testing (as appropriate per local clinic policy)	✔	✔	If further UPSI has taken place
Creatinine	✔	Only if abnormalities at baseline	
Alanine transaminase (ALT)	✔	Only if abnormalities at baseline, Hep B/C co-infected or on Kaletra	
Urinalysis or uPCR	✔	Only if abnormalities at baseline	If abnormalities at baseline or 2 weeks
Pregnancy test	✔	If appropriate	If appropriate

Adapted from *International Journal of STD & AIDS* 2016; April: doi: 10.1177/0956462416641813, with permission from SAGE.

Long-term psychological support may be needed for victims of sexual assault because anxiety and depression are common consequences. Therefore if an individual presents to a GUM or integrated sexual health service, letters are often sent to the individual's GP with the attendee's consent.

14.5.4 Pregnancy following assault

There is approximately a 5% risk of pregnancy following a sexual assault. For individuals not currently using contraception the need for emergency contraception should be considered (see *Chapter 13*). Pregnancy testing is undertaken no earlier than 3 weeks after the sexual assault.

• Assailant from high-risk group. • Background local prevalence of HIV in community. • HIV status of assailant (if known). • Assailant thought to come from a high prevalence area. • Type of assault.	• Assailant stranger versus known. • Presence of other STI(s) in the assaulted individual. • Genital injury. • Multiple assailants. • Multiple risk factors.

Figure 14.2. HIV risk factors.

Table 14.5. Situations when PEPSE is considered

	Source HIV status			
	HIV positive		**Unknown HIV status**	
	HIV viral load unknown / detectable (>200 copies/ml)	HIV viral load undetectable (<200 copies/ml)	From high prevalence country / risk group[1]	From low prevalence country / group
Receptive anal sex	Recommend	Not recommended[2] *Provided source has confirmed HIV viral load <200 c/ml for >6 months*	Recommend	Not recommended
Insertive anal sex	Recommend	Not recommended	Consider[3]	Not recommended
Receptive vaginal sex	Recommend	Not recommended	Consider[3]	Not recommended
Insertive vaginal sex	Consider[4]	Not recommended	Consider[3]	Not recommended
Fellatio with ejaculation[5]	Not recommended	Not recommended	Not recommended	Not recommended
Fellatio without ejaculation[5]	Not recommended	Not recommended	Not recommended	Not recommended

	Source HIV status			
	HIV positive		Unknown HIV status	
Splash of semen into eye	Not recommended	Not recommended	Not recommended	Not recommended
Cunnilingus	Not recommended	Not recommended	Not recommended	Not recommended
Sharing of injecting equipment[6]	Recommend	Not recommended	Consider	Not recommended
Human bite[7]	Not recommended	Not recommended	Not recommended	Not recommended
Needlestick from a discarded needle in the community			Not recommended	Not recommended

Reproduced from *International Journal of STD & AIDS* 2016; April; doi: 10.1177/0956462416641813 with permission from SAGE.

[1] High prevalence countries or risk groups are those where there is a significant likelihood of the source individual being HIV positive. Within the UK at present, this is likely to be men who have sex with men, intravenous drug users from high-risk countries (see footnote 6) and individuals who have immigrated to the UK from areas of high HIV prevalence, particularly sub-Saharan Africa (high prevalence is >1%). Country-specific HIV prevalence can be found in UNAIDS Gap Report: www.unaids. org/en/resources/campaigns/2014/2014gapreport/gapreport.

[2] The source's viral load must be confirmed with the source's clinic as <200 copies/ml for >6 months. Where there is any uncertainty about results or adherence to ART then PEPSE should be given after unprotected anal intercourse with an HIV-positive person.

[3] More detailed knowledge of local prevalence of HIV within communities may change these recommendations from Consider to Recommend in areas of particularly high HIV prevalence. Co-factors that influence the likelihood of transmission should be considered (see *Box 1* in the guidelines at www.bashh.org/documents/PEPSE%202015%20guideline%20final_NICE.pdf).

[4] Co-factors in *Box 1* that influence the likelihood of transmission should be considered.

[5] PEPSE is not recommended for individuals receiving fellatio i.e. inserting their penis into another's oral cavity. For individuals giving fellatio PEPSE is not recommended unless HIV seroconversion and/or oropharyngeal trauma / ulceration are present; see notes in guideline cited in footnote 3.

[6] HIV prevalence amongst intravenous drug users varies considerably depending on country of origin and is particularly high in those from eastern Europe and central Asia. Region-specific estimates can be found in the UNAIDS Gap Report: www.unaids.org/sites/default/files/media_asset/05_Peoplewhoinjectdrugs.pdf.

[7] A bite is assumed to constitute breakage of the skin with passage of blood. See notes in guideline cited in footnote 3 about extreme circumstances where PEP could be considered after discussion with a specialist.

EXAMPLE

A 28 year old school receptionist attends for a contraception discussion at her GPs. She states she has no symptoms but she ended the relationship with her partner of 2 years about a month ago when she discovered he has another sexual partner.

Which questions are you going to ask her? Which investigations are you going to offer and when will you need to repeat any of the investigations?

1. Ask about potential symptoms, including change in vaginal discharge, dysuria, abdominal or pelvic pain, skin changes. Also ask about menstrual history, including last menstrual period, intermenstrual or post-coital bleeding. Ask about current contraception and condom use, previous sexual partner(s), history of previous STIs and blood-borne virus risk assessment.
2. Offer physical examination even in absence of symptoms because infection with, for example, genital warts may be identified.
3. Screening of vagina with NAAT for chlamydia and gonorrhoea, and clotted blood for HIV and syphilis form the main components of a routine asymptomatic screen. If the last sexual contact was more than 3 months ago no further testing will be required. In this particular case HIV and syphilis testing should be repeated 3 months after the last sexual contact.

References

BASHH (2008) *UK National Guidelines for HIV Testing*. BHIVA, BASSH, BIF
  [available at www.bashh.org – accessed April 2016]

BASHH (2012a) *UK National Guidelines on Safer Sex Advice*. Clinical Effectiveness Group BASHH and BHIVA.
  [available at www.bashh.org – accessed April 2016]

BASHH (2012b) *UK National Guidelines on the Management of Adult and Adolescent Complainants of Sexual Assault*. Clinical Effectiveness Group
  [available at www.bashh.org – accessed April 2016]

BASHH (2015) *Summary Guidance on Test for Sexually Transmitted Infection*. Clinical Effectiveness Group.
  [available at www.bashh.org – accessed April 2016]

BASHH (2015) *UK Guideline for the Use of HIV Post-Exposure Prophylaxis Following Sexual Exposure (PEPSE)*
  [www.bashh.org/documents/PEPSE%202015%20guideline%20final_NICE.pdf – accessed April 2016]

EAGA (2014) *Guidance on HIV post-exposure prophylaxis*, Expert Advisory Group on AIDS
  [www.gov.uk/government/publications/eaga-guidance-on-hiv-post-exposure-prophylaxis – accessed April 2016]

Chapter 15
Unplanned pregnancy

15.1 Introduction

Recent research suggests that 1 in 6 pregnancies in Britain are unplanned, with 1 in 60 women experiencing an unplanned pregnancy in any given year.

For some women discovering they are pregnant is an exciting, highly anticipated event. For others it can be associated with mixed emotions including:
- shock that they are actually pregnant
- concern about the responsibility associated with being pregnant
- fear that they are not ready, or are unable to afford a child (or another child)
- anger that they did not choose to be pregnant
- anxiety about being pregnant or what others will think of the pregnancy
- concern that they need to make a decision about the pregnancy and fear they will make the wrong decision
- negative associations with the conception and/or father, particularly in the case of the victims of sexual assault.

As no method of contraception is 100% effective, the provision of services to facilitate the management of an unplanned pregnancy is an important component of any contraception and sexual health service.

Support and the provision of information are available for women who find that they are pregnant and are not sure what to do. The options include:
- continuing with the pregnancy and keeping the baby, or putting the baby up for fostering or adoption
- ending the pregnancy with an abortion.

Discussion with family members, friends, medical and nursing professionals and charitable organizations can provide support and information to facilitate the decision-making process.

15.2 Adoption

- Adoption is an option for women who do not want to keep the baby but do not wish or are too late to have an abortion.
- The process of adoption is organized by adoption agencies and local authorities.
- An adoption is a legal process and once the process is complete it cannot be undone.
- The formal agreement for the adoption is signed once the baby is six weeks old. Up until this time the child will usually live with foster carers while arrangements are made for adoption. After this, the child is placed in the care of the adoptive parents who make an application to the court for an adoption order which makes them the child's legal parents. The child lives with the adoptive parents for 13 weeks before they can apply through the court to make the adoption legal.
- The British Association of Adoption and Fostering (www.baaf.org.uk) can provide useful information and local contacts.

15.3 Abortion

- Legal abortion is a safe way to end a pregnancy. It is the most common gynaecological procedure undertaken in Great Britain and by the age of 45 one-third of women will have had an abortion. See *Section 15.7* for the legal situation in Ireland.
- Within England, Wales and Scotland the rate of abortion in those under the age of 18 is declining.
- Just over 90% of abortions are carried out when the pregnancy is under 13 completed weeks of gestation.
- Although the structure of abortion services varies from area to area, all women considering this option should have access to care and services of a uniformly high quality.
- Under the current commissioning structure, abortions are commissioned by clinical commissioning groups. A full range of services including a choice of medical and surgical procedures for all gestations, up to the legal limit of 24 weeks of gestation, should be provided either directly or through a referral pathway.
- Services are provided by the NHS or independent providers such as Marie Stopes International (MSI) or British Pregnancy Advisory Service (BPAS). In accordance with the 1967 Abortion Act, an abortion can only be carried out in locations approved by the Secretary of State for Health.
- Generally abortion services are widely accessible and take referrals from a number of sources including general practitioners, sexual health services and self-referral (ideally via a centralized telephone system).
- Once a woman makes the decision she would like to proceed with an abortion there should be minimal delay. An initial assessment appointment is ideally offered within 5 working days of referral. The time from initially seeing the provider and making a decision to the abortion taking place should not exceed 10 days. Collectively, from referral to procedure the process should take less than 21 days.

- Importantly a woman can cancel or delay appointments or the procedure at any point if she wishes to.

15.3.1 Pre-abortion assessment

- Within the consultation the following should be documented:
  - reasons why the unplanned pregnancy may have occurred and why the woman is requesting an abortion
  - details of the past menstrual history, including last menstrual period and cycle
  - previous contraceptive methods used and problems with these methods
  - contraceptive plans for the future
  - past medical history, including obstetric history
  - social and relationship history, with particular reference to domestic violence and safeguarding issues.
- Pregnancy should be confirmed. Although an ultrasound scan is not essential it is increasingly being used to assess gestation and to confirm that the pregnancy is within the uterine cavity.
- Discuss pregnancy options, including fostering and adoption.
- Identify women who require more support in the decision-making process.
- Methods of abortion should be discussed and the procedures explained, including potential adverse effects and complications. This should be supported by written information.
- STI screening should be undertaken in at-risk groups along with standard assessment of VTE risk and rhesus status.
- Finally, consent for the chosen procedure is obtained and, in the UK, the HSA1 form is completed by two doctors indicating in good faith the grounds for performing the abortion (see *Figure 15.1*). It is not legally essential for either or both doctors to see the patient before the HSA1 form is completed; however, they must review each case and document in the clinical notes the grounds for performing the abortion. **C** is the most common ground for performing an abortion (see *Table 15.1*).

A	Continuance of the pregnancy would involve risk to the life of the pregnant woman greater than if the pregnancy were terminated
B	Termination is necessary to prevent grave permanent injury to the physical or mental health of the pregnant woman
C	The pregnancy has NOT exceeded its 24th week and continuance of the pregnancy would involve risk, greater than if the pregnancy were terminated, of injury to the physical or mental health of the pregnant woman
D	The pregnancy has NOT exceeded its 24th week and continuance of the pregnancy would involve risk, greater than if the pregnancy were terminated, of injury to the physical or mental health of any existing child(ren) of the family of the pregnant woman
E	There is a substantial risk that if the child were born it would suffer from such physical or mental abnormalities as to be seriously handicapped

Figure 15.1. Grounds for abortion in the UK.

15.3.2 Abortion procedures

- Providers should ideally give a choice of medical and surgical abortion, irrespective of gestation.
- The options for method of abortion are determined by gestation and the wishes of the woman in attendance (see *Figure 15.2*).
- While the majority of procedures are undertaken as day cases, certain circumstances such as medical problems, social indications, geographical factors or individual choice may necessitate an in-patient stay.

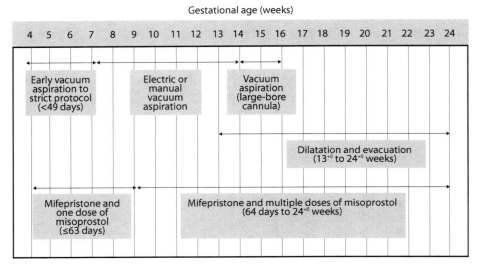

Gestational age (weeks)

Figure 15.2. Summary of abortion methods appropriate for use in abortion services in the UK by gestational age (in weeks). Figure reproduced with permission from the Royal College of Obstetricians and Gynaecologists.

Medical abortion

Medical abortion (with mifepristone and misoprostol) is *licensed* for the provision of abortion up to 9 weeks and from 13 weeks to 23 weeks and 6 days. However, in practice it is provided through all gestations. Medical abortions are commenced within a hospital or clinic setting, but in early gestations may end in an individual's home.

- Medical abortion is a two-stage process:
  - initially, 200 mg of mifepristone is administered orally; it is a steroid with a similar structure to progesterone and blocks the action of progesterone on the uterus and sensitizes the uterus to prostaglandin
  - 24–48 hours after the first stage, misoprostol (800 mcg) is administered orally, vaginally or sublingually; it causes uterine contraction and expulsion of the products of conception
- In later gestations, further doses of misoprostol (400 mcg) may be administered at 3-hourly intervals, to a maximum of four additional doses.

- After misoprostol has been administered, women below 9 weeks of gestation can either:
  - remain in hospital or clinic until the products of conception are seen, or
  - remain for a short time to ensure no adverse reactions occur, then go home and pass the products of conception there, with follow-up to ensure the procedure is complete and the pregnancy is not ongoing.
- Above 21 weeks of gestation, the abortion is preceded by fetocide, most commonly achieved by injecting potassium chloride under ultrasound guidance.
- Early medical abortion (before 9 weeks of gestation) is very effective, with a failure rate of less than 1 in 200.
- Symptoms experienced during medical abortion include cramping abdominal pain, bleeding, nausea, vomiting, diarrhoea, flushes and sweats and dizziness.

Surgical abortion

Surgical abortion can be carried out at all gestations up to 23 weeks and 6 days of gestation:
- a suction termination can be performed up to 13 weeks
- dilatation and evacuation (D&E) of the uterus is carried out in larger gestations because the products are too large to be removed intact through the cervix and are therefore removed piecemeal; this is normally performed under ultrasound guidance.

Under 13 weeks of gestation, there are potentially two methods of surgical abortion depending on local availability.
- Manual vacuum aspiration (MVA) is performed under local anaesthetic or conscious sedation. A plastic cannula is introduced through the cervix and an aspirator attached. The vacuum is released and uterine evacuation accomplished.
- Electronic vacuum aspiration (EVA) is performed under general anaesthetic. Appropriate cervical dilatation is undertaken, with graduated dilators if needed, then the suction curette is introduced through the cervix and suction applied; the products are removed in a closed system until complete evacuation of the uterus is achieved.

Cervical priming, for example 400 mcg of misoprostol vaginally or orally, is considered prior to all cases because it reduces the risk of cervical trauma and for MVA may remove the need for dilatation.

15.3.3 Following the abortion

- Irrespective of the method used, following an abortion prophylactic antibiotics are normally prescribed to reduce the risk of post-abortion infection. The antibiotics provided are typically metronidazole 1 g rectally and azithromycin 1 g orally, or doxycycline 100 mg twice a day for 7 days.
- Rhesus status is determined prior to abortion and rhesus-negative women are given anti-D IgG immunoprophylaxis within 72 hours of the abortion.
- In the UK an HSA4 form is completed by the practitioner undertaking the abortion, either online or as a paper copy, and this is sent to the Chief Medical Officer within 14 days of the abortion.
- Fetal remains should always be managed respectfully. Disposal is by cremation or burial and is generally organized by the hospital or clinic performing the abortion.

15.4 Complications

Abortion is a safe procedure with major complications rare at all gestations (see *Table 15.2*). Estimated complication rates are 1–2 per 1000 abortions. It is difficult to truly determine the rate, partly due to lack of standardization of reporting criteria and partly because women experiencing complications often present to other healthcare providers.

Table 15.2. Complications of surgical and medical abortion

Complication	Rate
Uterine perforation (surgical only)	1–4 per 1000
Haemorrhage	1–4 per 1000
Cervix trauma (surgical only)	<1 per 100
Infection	1 per 10
Retained products of conception	<5 per 100
Failure of procedure to end pregnancy	<1 per 100
Anaesthetic	Rare
Psychological consequences	Currently not quantified
Infertility	No proven association

15.5 Post-abortion contraception

Provision of contraception immediately following abortion is key to reducing further unplanned pregnancies. Wherever possible the chosen method should be started immediately following the abortion. Where the requested method is not available a bridging method can be provided.

- Most contraceptive methods including CHC, POP, injectable, implant and IUC can be started immediately or soon after a medical or surgical abortion.
- A diaphragm can be fitted 4–6 weeks after abortion.
- Sterilization is ideally undertaken 3 months or so after an abortion to allow time to consider this permanent choice.

Ideally, if all methods of contraception are not available within the abortion service, referral pathways to local sexual health services/general practitioners will be in place.

15.6 Aftercare

- After an abortion a 24-hour telephone number should be provided to women so that they can access help or discuss any concerns.
- Women should contact abortion services or their general practitioner post-procedure if they have a temperature, have persisting abdominal pain, prolonged heavy bleeding, abdominal tenderness or abnormal vaginal discharge.
- Women are generally advised that routine follow-up is not needed. Pregnancy symptoms resolve within 3 days of the abortion and their next period will occur within 4–6 weeks.

15.7 Legal situation in Ireland

15.7.1 Northern Ireland

Abortion is legal in Northern Ireland in some circumstances. However, most women have to travel to England although they are not entitled to an NHS abortion in England. The 1945 Criminal Justice (Northern Ireland) Act allows the abortion of a "child capable of being born alive" only where the mother's life would otherwise be put at risk. In 2003 after judicial review, Mr Justice Kerr stated that abortion is legal in Northern Ireland if:

- continuance of the pregnancy threatens the life of the mother, or would adversely affect her mental or physical health
- the adverse effect on her mental or physical health must be a "real and serious" one, and must also be "permanent or long-term"
- in most cases, the risk of the adverse effect occurring would need to be a probability, but a possibility might be regarded as sufficient if the imminent death of the mother was the potential adverse effect
- it will always be a question of fact and degree whether the perceived effect of a non-termination is sufficiently grave to warrant terminating the pregnancy in a particular case.

The above guidance is ambiguous and a guidance document from the Department of Health, Social Services and Public Safety is still awaited.

15.7.2 Republic of Ireland

Before 2013, abortion was illegal in the Republic of Ireland unless it occurred as the result of a medical intervention performed to save the life of the mother. In 2012 more than 4000 women travelled to the UK to obtain help. In 2013 a new Act was passed: 'Protection of Life During Pregnancy Act 2013'.

- Within this legal document there is a single offence of the intentional destruction of "unborn human life" with a maximum sentence being reduced from life imprisonment to 14 years.
- However, the 2013 Act states that abortion is legal when there is a real and substantial risk to a woman's life (including risk brought about by a threat of suicide), and where the procedures carried out in the Act are complied with.

15.8 Myths and misconceptions

- **You will not be able to become pregnant again after having an abortion** – this is not true. Well-designed studies show no connection between abortion and future fertility problems. There is less evidence investigating repeat or second-trimester abortion but current research indicates no association in the absence of complications.
- **Abortions can weaken the cervix making premature delivery of a baby more common following such a procedure** – this is not true. There was a link 20–30 years ago when there was a 10–20% increased risk, but with modern abortion methods (particularly medical) abortion data from 2000 onwards show no association of premature delivery in subsequent pregnancies.

- **Abortions cause long-term psychological harm for most women** – there is no well-conducted research to support this. Women with an unwanted pregnancy are at risk of mental health problems, but a woman with an unwanted pregnancy is equally as likely to have mental health problems from experiencing an abortion as she is from giving birth.

EXAMPLE

A 19 year old attends your practice with a positive pregnancy test. Her last period was 7 weeks ago.

What additional information would you need and what are her options?

1. Is the pregnancy planned and how does she feel about being pregnant?
2. Document details of menstrual cycle, current contraception, medical history and social history.
3. Discuss all options available, including continuing with the pregnancy and keeping the baby or placing the child in foster care or for adoption, or abortion.
4. If abortion is requested by this 19 year old, referral/self-referral to an abortion service should be expedited. At this clinic an assessment is undertaken.
5. Both medical and surgical abortion may be discussed and the most appropriate method selected as long as no contraindications to medical abortion are identified, such as severe asthma, long-term steroid use, renal or hepatic failure or cardiovascular disease.
6. Contraception after abortion should be covered pre-abortion and commenced immediately after the procedure or with minimal delay.

References

Department of Health (2014) *Guidance in Relation to Requirements of the Abortion Act 1967*
[www.gov.uk/government/uploads/system/uploads/attachment_data/file/313459/20140509_-_Abortion_Guidance_Document.pdf – accessed April 2016]

Department of Health (2015) *Abortion statistics, England and Wales: 2015*
[www.gov.uk/government/statistics/report-on-abortion-statistics-in-england-and-wales-for-2015 – accessed June 2016]

Gov.uk (2014) *Child Adoption*
[www.gov.uk/child-adoption/overview – accessed April 2016]

RCOG (2011) *The Care of Women Requesting Induced Abortion* (Evidence-based Guideline Number 7)
[www.rcog.org.uk/globalassets/documents/guidelines/abortion-guideline_web_1.pdf – accessed April 2016]

Appendix

Summary of the UKMEC for contraceptive use

UKMEC Categories:

1 = no restriction for use

2 = can generally be used but with careful follow-up

3 = not usually recommended but may be used after expert clinical judgement and/or referral to a contraceptive specialist

4 = use poses an unacceptable health risk

UKMEC SUMMARY TABLE HORMONAL AND INTRAUTERINE CONTRACEPTION
Cu-IUD = Copper-bearing intrauterine device; LNG-IUS = Levonorgestrel-releasing intrauterine system; IMP = Progestogen-only implant; DMPA = Progestogen-only injectable: depot medroxyprogesterone acetate; POP = Progestogen-only pill; CHC = Combined hormonal contraception

CONDITION	Cu-IUD	LNG-IUS	IMP	DMPA	POP	CHC
	I = Initiation, C = Continuation					
PERSONAL CHARACTERISTICS AND REPRODUCTIVE HISTORY						
Pregnancy	NA	NA	NA	NA	NA	NA
Age	Menarche to <20=2, ≥20=1	Menarche to <20=2, ≥20=1	After menarche = 1	Menarche to <18=2, 18–45=1, >45=2	After menarche = 1	Menarche to <40=1, ≥40=2
Parity						
a) Nulliparous	1	1	1	1	1	1
b) Parous	1	1	1	1	1	1
Breastfeeding						
a) 0 to <6 weeks postpartum	See below		1	2	1	4
b) ≥6 weeks to <6 months (primarily breastfeeding)	See below		1	1	1	2
c) ≥6 months postpartum	See below		1	1	1	1
Postpartum (in non-breastfeeding women)						
a) 0 to <3 weeks						
(i) With other risk factors for VTE	See below		1	2	1	4
(ii) Without other risk factors	See below		1	2	1	3
b) 3 to <6 weeks						
(i) With other risk factors for VTE	See below		1	2	1	3
(ii) Without other risk factors	See below		1	1	1	2
c) ≥6 weeks			1	1	1	1
Postpartum (in breastfeeding or non-breastfeeding women, including post-Caesarean section)						
a) 0 to <48 hours	1	1	See above			
b) 48 hours to <4 weeks	3	3	See above			
c) ≥4 weeks	1	1	See above			
d) Postpartum sepsis	4	4	See above			

CONDITION	Cu-IUD	LNG-IUS	IMP	DMPA	POP	CHC
	I = Initiation, C = Continuation					
Post-abortion						
a) First trimester	1	1	1	1	1	1
b) Second trimester	2	2	1	1	1	1
c) Post-abortion sepsis	4	4	1	1	1	1
Past ectopic pregnancy	1	1	1	1	1	1
History of pelvic surgery (see postpartum, including Caesarean section)	1	1	1	1	1	1
Smoking						
a) Age <35 years	1	1	1	1	1	2
b) Age ≥35 years						
(i) <15 cigarettes/day	1	1	1	1	1	3
(ii) ≥15 cigarettes/day	1	1	1	1	1	4
(iii) Stopped smoking <1 year	1	1	1	1	1	3
(iv) Stopped smoking ≥1 year	1	1	1	1	1	2
Obesity						
a) BMI ≥30–34 kg/m²	1	1	1	1	1	2
b) BMI ≥35 kg/m²	1	1	1	1	1	3
History of bariatric surgery	The following bold entries are additions to the UKMEC in 2016					
a) With BMI <30 kg/m²	**1**	**1**	**1**	**1**	**1**	**1**
b) With BMI ≥30–34 kg/m²	**1**	**1**	**1**	**1**	**1**	**2**
c) With BMI ≥35 kg/m²	**1**	**1**	**1**	**1**	**1**	**3**
Organ transplant						
a) Complicated: graft failure (acute or chronic), rejection, cardiac allograft vasculopathy	I 3 / C 2	I 3 / C 2	**2**	**2**	**2**	**3**
b) Uncomplicated	**2**	**2**	**2**	**2**	**2**	**2**
CARDIOVASCULAR DISEASE (CVD)						
Multiple risk factors for CVD (such as smoking, diabetes, hypertension, obesity and dyslipidaemias)	1	2	2	3	2	3
Hypertension						
a) Adequately controlled hypertension	1	1	1	2	1	3

CONDITION	Cu-IUD	LNG-IUS		IMP		DMPA	POP		CHC
		I = Initiation, C = Continuation							
b) Consistently elevated BP levels (properly taken measurements)									
(i) Systolic >140–159 mmHg or diastolic >90–99 mmHg	1	1		1		1	1		3
(ii) Systolic ≥160 mmHg or diastolic ≥100 mmHg	1	1		1		2	1		4
c) Vascular disease	1	2		2		3	2		4
History of high BP during pregnancy	1	1		1		1	1		2
Current and history of ischaemic heart disease	1	I: 2	C: 3	I: 2	C: 3	3	I: 2	C: 3	4
Stroke (history of cerebrovascular accident, including TIA)	1	I: 2	C: 3	I: 2	C: 3	3	I: 2	C: 3	4
Known dyslipidaemias	1	2		2		2	2		2
Venous thromboembolism (VTE)									
a) History of VTE	1	2		2		2	2		4
b) Current VTE (on anticoagulants)	1	2		2		2	2		4
c) Family history of VTE									
(i) First-degree relative age <45 years	1	1		1		1	1		3
(ii) First-degree relative age ≥45 years	1	1		1		1	1		2
d) Major surgery									
(i) With prolonged immobilisation	1	2		2		2	2		4
(ii) Without prolonged immobilisation	1	1		1		1	1		2
e) Minor surgery without immobilisation	1	1		1		1	1		1
f) Immobility (unrelated to surgery) (e.g. wheelchair use, debilitating illness)	1	1		1		1	1		3
Superficial venous thrombosis									
a) Varicose veins	1	1		1		1	1		1
b) Superficial venous thrombosis	1	1		1		1	1		2

CONDITION	Cu-IUD	LNG-IUS	IMP	DMPA	POP	CHC
	I = Initiation, C = Continuation					
Known thrombogenic mutations (e.g. factor V Leiden, prothrombin mutation, protein S, protein C and antithrombin deficiencies)	1	2	2	2	2	4
Valvular and congenital heart disease						
a) Uncomplicated	1	1	1	1	1	2
b) Complicated (e.g. pulmonary hypertension, history of subacute bacterial endocarditis)	2	2	1	1	1	4
Cardiomyopathy	The following bold entries are additions to the UKMEC in 2016					
a) Normal cardiac function	**1**	**1**	**1**	**1**	**1**	**2**
b) Impaired cardiac function	**2**	**2**	**2**	**2**	**2**	**4**
Cardiac arrhythmias						
a) Atrial fibrillation	**1**	**2**	**2**	**2**	**2**	**4**
b) Known long QT syndrome	I 3 / C 1	I 3 / C 1	**1**	**2**	**1**	**2**
NEUROLOGICAL CONDITIONS						
Headaches						
a) Non-migrainous (mild or severe)	1	1	1	1	1	I 1 / C 2
b) Migraine without aura, at any age	1	2	2	2	I 1 / C 2	I 2 / C 3
c) Migraine with aura, at any age	1	2	2	2	2	4
d) History (≥5 years ago) of migraine with aura, any age	1	2	2	2	2	3
Idiopathic intracranial hypertension (IIH)	1	1	1	1	1	2
Epilepsy	1	1	1	1	1	1
Taking anti-epileptic drugs	Certain anti-epileptic drugs have the potential to affect the bioavailability of steroid hormones in hormonal contraception. For up-to-date information on the potential drug interactions between hormonal contraception and anti-epileptic drugs, please refer to the online drug interaction checker available on the Medscape website (http://reference.medscape.com/drug-interactionchecker).					
DEPRESSIVE DISORDERS						

CONDITION	Cu-IUD		LNG-IUS		IMP	DMPA	POP	CHC	
	I = Initiation, C = Continuation								
Depressive disorders	1		1		1	1	1	1	
BREAST AND REPRODUCTIVE TRACT CONDITIONS									
Vaginal bleeding patterns									
a) Irregular pattern without heavy bleeding	1		1		2	2	2	1	
b) Heavy or prolonged bleeding (includes regular and irregular patterns)	2		I: 1	C: 2	2	2	2	1	
Unexplained vaginal bleeding (suspicious for serious condition) before evaluation	I: 4	C: 2	I: 4	C: 2	3	3	2	2	
Endometriosis	2		1		1	1	1	1	
Benign ovarian tumours (including cysts)	1		1		1	1	1	1	
Severe dysmenorrhoea	2		1		1	1	1	1	
Gestational trophoblastic disease (GTD)									
a) Undetectable hCG levels	1		1		1	1	1	1	
b) Decreasing hCG levels	3		3		1	1	1	1	
c) Persistently elevated hCG levels or malignant disease	4		4		1	1	1	1	
Cervical ectropion	1		1		1	1	1	1	
Cervical intraepithelial neoplasia (CIN)	1		2		1	2	1	2	
Cervical cancer									
a) Awaiting treatment	I: 4	C: 2	I: 4	C: 2	2	2	1	2	
b) Radical trachelectomy	3		3		2	2	1	2	
Breast conditions									
a) Undiagnosed mass/breast symptoms	1		2		2	2	2	I: 3	C: 2
b) Benign breast conditions	1		1		1	1	1	1	
c) Family history of breast cancer	1		1		1	1	1	1	
d) Carriers of known gene mutations associated with breast cancer (e.g. BRCA1/BRCA2)	1		2		2	2	2	3	
e) Breast cancer									
(i) Current breast cancer	1		4		4	4	4	4	

CONDITION	Cu-IUD		LNG-IUS		IMP	DMPA	POP	CHC
	I = Initiation, C = Continuation							
(ii) Past breast cancer	1		3		3	3	3	3
Endometrial cancer	**I**	**C**	**I**	**C**	1	1	1	1
	4	2	4	2				
Ovarian cancer	1		1		1	1	1	1
Uterine fibroids								
a) Without distortion of the uterine cavity	1		1		1	1	1	1
b) With distortion of the uterine cavity	3		3		1	1	1	1
Anatomical abnormalities								
a) Distorted uterine cavity	3		3					
b) Other abnormalities	2		2					
Pelvic inflammatory disease (PID)								
a) Past PID (assuming no current risk factor for STIs)	1		1		1	1	1	1
b) Current PID	**I**	**C**	**I**	**C**	1	1	1	1
	4	2	4	2				
Sexually transmitted infections (STIs)								
a) Chlamydial infection (current)	**I**	**C**	**I**	**C**				
(i) Symptomatic	4	2	4	2	1	1	1	1
(ii) Asymptomatic	3	2	3	2	1	1	1	1
b) Purulent cervicitis or gonorrhoea (current)	4	2	4	2	1	1	1	1
c) Other current STIs (excluding HIV & hepatitis)	2		2		1	1	1	1
d) Vaginitis (including *Trichomonas vaginalis* and bacterial vaginosis) (current)	2		2		1	1	1	1
e) Increased risk for STIs	2		2		1	1	1	1
HIV INFECTION								
HIV infection								
a) High risk of HIV infection	2		2		1	1	1	1
b) HIV infected								
(i) CD4 count ≥200 cells/mm³	2		2		1	1	1	1
(ii) CD4 count <200 cells/mm³	**I**	**C**	**I**	**C**	1	1	1	1
	3	2	3	2				

CONDITION	Cu-IUD	LNG-IUS	IMP	DMPA	POP	CHC
	I = Initiation, C = Continuation					
c) Taking antiretroviral (ARV) drugs	Certain ARV drugs have the potential to affect the bioavailability of steroid hormones in hormonal contraception. For up-to-date information on the potential drug interactions between hormonal contraception and ARV drugs, please refer to the online HIV drugs interaction checker (www.hiv-druginteractions.org/interactions.aspx).					
OTHER INFECTIONS						
Tuberculosis						
a) Non-pelvic	1	1	1	1	1	1
b) Pelvic	I 4 / C 3	I 4 / C 3	1	1	1	1
ENDOCRINE CONDITIONS						
Diabetes						
a) History of gestational disease	1	1	1	1	1	1
b) Non-vascular disease						
(i) Non-insulin dependent	1	2	2	2	2	2
(ii) Insulin dependent	1	2	2	2	2	2
c) Nephropathy/retinopathy/ neuropathy	1	2	2	2	2	3
d) Other vascular disease	1	2	2	2	2	3
Thyroid disorders						
a) Simple goitre	1	1	1	1	1	1
b) Hyperthyroid	1	1	1	1	1	1
c) Hypothyroid	1	1	1	1	1	1
GASTROINTESTINAL CONDITIONS						
Gallbladder disease						
a) Symptomatic						
(i) Treated by cholecystectomy	1	2	2	2	2	2
(ii) Medically treated	1	2	2	2	2	3
(iii) Current	1	2	2	2	2	3
b) Asymptomatic	1	2	2	2	2	2
History of cholestasis						
a) Pregnancy related	1	1	1	1	1	2
b) Past COC related	1	2	2	2	2	3
Viral hepatitis						
a) Acute or flare	1	1	1	1	1	I 3 / C 2
b) Carrier	1	1	1	1	1	1

CONDITION	Cu-IUD	LNG-IUS	IMP	DMPA	POP	CHC
	I = Initiation, C = Continuation					
c) Chronic	1	1	1	1	1	1
Cirrhosis						
a) Mild (compensated without complications)	1	1	1	1	1	1
b) Severe (decompensated)	1	3	3	3	3	4
Liver tumours						
a) Benign						
(i) Focal nodular hyperplasia	1	2	2	2	2	2
(ii) Hepatocellular adenoma	1	3	3	3	3	4
b) Malignant (hepatocellular carcinoma)	1	3	3	3	3	4
Inflammatory bowel disease (including Crohn's disease and ulcerative colitis)	1	1	1	1	2	2
ANAEMIAS						
Thalassaemia	2	1	1	1	1	1
Sickle cell disease	2	1	1	1	1	2
Iron deficiency anaemia	2	1	1	1	1	1
RHEUMATIC DISEASES						
Rheumatoid arthritis	**1**	**2**	**2**	**2**	**2**	**2**
Systemic lupus erythematosus (SLE)						
a) No antiphospholipid antibodies	1	2	2	2	2	2
b) Positive antiphospholipid antibodies	1	2	2	2	2	4
Positive antiphospholipid antibodies	1	2	2	2	2	4
DRUG INTERACTIONS						
Taking medication	See section on drug interactions with hormonal contraception.					

Note: **Bold** entries in this table indicate changes to the UKMEC in 2016.

Index

Bold indicates main entry
Italic indicates a figure or table